ABC OF
COMPLEMENTARY MEDICINE

CATHERINE ZOLLMAN

General Practitioner, Bristol, UK

and

ANDREW J VICKERS

Memorial Sloan-Kettering Cancer Center, New York, USA

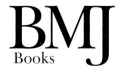

BMJ
Books

© BMJ Books 2000
BMJ Books is an imprint of the BMJ Publishing Group

First published in 2000
by BMJ Books, BMA House, Tavistock Square,
London WC1H 9JR

www.bmjbooks.com

British Library Cataloguing in Publication Data
A catalogue record for this book is available from the British Library

ISBN 0-7279-1237-2

Composition by Scribe Design, Gillingham, Kent
Printed and bound in Italy

615 5 20c Q 12.46

ABC OF
COMPLEMENTARY MEDICINE

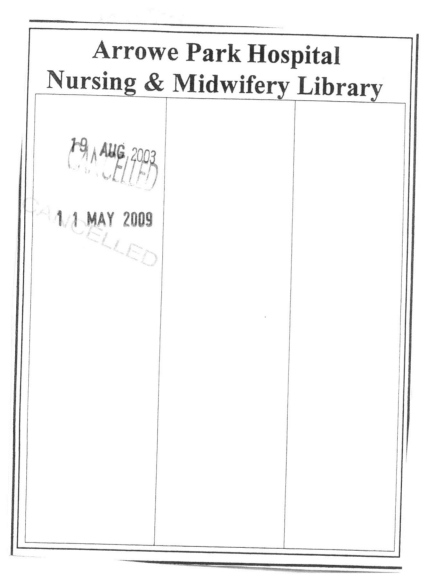

Contents

Preface

Recent trends in the provision and public usage of complementary medicine dictate that conventionally trained health professionals now need to be conversant with the main complementary therapies. This is so that they can remain informed and centrally involved in their patients' healthcare. Our aim in publishing this *ABC of Complementary Medicine* has been to bring together appropriate information in a way that doctors and other professionals will find both relevant and practical.

Throughout the text our over-arching objectives have been: clarity and comprehensibility; accuracy (including making it clear which statements are based on research evidence, which on clinical experience and which on theoretical considerations); and as much objectivity as the human condition permits. Each chapter has been thoroughly peer reviewed by medical and non-medical complementary therapy practitioners and researchers.

We recognise that most doctors will never have received any formal education in this field, and that many may even be uncertain about the precise meaning of the term complementary medicine. This is not surprising since over the last few years there have been many changes and many confusing, ambiguous, and overlapping terminologies have been used. One of our main aims has been to emphasise that *complementary medicine* is a catch-all category that includes a large number of disparate practices. However, we have also attempted to capture something of the essence of complementary medicine as a whole, and explore the respects in which it is similar to and different from conventional medical practice. Thus our articles cover issues such as the theoretical basis, research evidence, historical context and training and regulation of various complementary disciplines, as well as ideas of holism, self-healing and the therapeutic relationship. Some of the ideas and theories presented may seem quite alien to a mind trained initially in the basic sciences, so we have tried to avoid complementary jargon and have focused instead on practical applications rather than theoretical detail.

The size and scope of this ABC means that it is very much what its title suggests, an introduction. The book should provide a rough working framework for the medical practitioner without any detailed knowledge of complementary medicine. The format does not allow for extensive references to the research literature, something that is problematic in such a scientifically controversial field. Accordingly, we provide sources of further reading and information for those who want to explore the subject in more depth.

The book is divided into three sections. The first three chapters provide a general introduction to complementary medicine. The first explores what is meant by *complementary medicine*, describing the range of disciplines which fall within this category and some of the features they have in common. The second chapter examines the use of complementary medicine by the public and by conventional health practitioners, reviewing survey and qualitative data on prevalence, behaviour and motivation. The third chapter, which focuses on the UK, explores the way in which complementary medical services are provided, particularly with reference to the National Health Service.

Chapters 4 to 10 deal with 7 of the main types of complementary therapies. For each discipline we provide a brief historical and philosophical background, describe what a treatment or consultation typically involves for patients, summarise the relevant research evidence and highlight important safety issues. Regulatory and training structures within each discipline are described and listed. This format was chosen to address both the concerns most commonly expressed by doctors and the questions most commonly asked by patients.

The last two chapters deal with some of the practical issues that complementary medicine raises for patients and doctors. These include the potential non-specific benefits (placebo) and problems (nocebo), as well as issues of control and communication

We recognise that in trying to present an introduction to such a wide and complex field there have been inevitable omissions and we may have appeared simplistic or over-general in places. This is, unfortunately, one of the inherent constraints of an ABC series. The publication in journal (particularly electronic) form has generated much discussion. Perhaps predictably, with a subject which is as emotive and broad ranging as this one, comments span the full spectrum of attitudes and, as authors, we hope that this stimulation of debate and airing of views will of itself encourage a better understanding between the worlds of conventional and complementary medicine. In time, we hope we will have contributed to establishing more clearly the way each can be used most appropriately within health care as a whole.

Catherine Zollman, Andrew Vickers
January 2000

Acknowledgement: We would like to take this opportunity to thank all of those who helped in the preparation of this series, particularly Trish Groves, Greg Cotton and Jan Croot of the *BMJ*.

1 What is complementary medicine?

Definitions and terms

Complementary medicine refers to a group of therapeutic and diagnostic disciplines that exist largely outside the institutions where conventional health care is taught and provided. Complementary medicine is an increasing feature of healthcare practice, but considerable confusion remains about what exactly it is and what position the disciplines included under this term should hold in relation to conventional medicine

In the 1970s and 1980s these disciplines were mainly provided as an alternative to conventional health care and hence became known collectively as "alternative medicine." The name "complementary medicine" developed as the two systems began to be used alongside (to "complement") each other. Over the years, "complementary" has changed from describing this relation between unconventional healthcare disciplines and conventional care to defining the group of disciplines itself. Some authorities use the term "unconventional medicine" synonymously. This changing and overlapping terminology may explain some of the confusion that surrounds the subject.

We use the term complementary medicine to describe healthcare practices such as those listed in the box. We use it synonymously with the terms "complementary therapies" and "complementary and alternative medicine" found in other texts, according to the definition used by the Cochrane Collaboration.

Which disciplines are complementary?

Our list is not exhaustive, and new branches of established disciplines are continually being developed. Also, what is thought to be conventional varies between countries and changes over time. The boundary between complementary and conventional medicine is therefore blurred and constantly shifting. For example, although osteopathy and chiropractic are still generally considered complementary therapies in Britain, they are included as part of standard care in guidelines from conventional bodies such as the Royal College of General Practitioners.

The wide range of disciplines classified as complementary medicine makes it difficult to find defining criteria that are common to all. Many of the assumptions made about complementary medicine are oversimplistic generalisations.

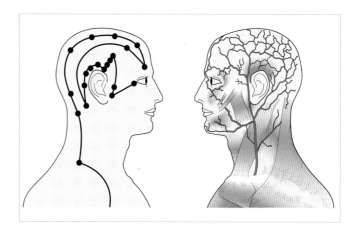

Common complementary therapies

- Acupressure
- Acupuncture*
- Alexander technique
- Applied kinesiology
- Anthroposophic medicine
- Aromatherapy*
- Autogenic training
- Ayurveda
- Chiropractic*
- Cranial osteopathy
- Environmental medicine
- Healing
- Herbal medicine*
- Homoeopathy*
- Hypnosis*
- Massage*
- Meditation*
- Naturopathy
- Nutritional therapy*
- Osteopathy*
- Reflexology*
- Reiki
- Relaxation and visualisation*
- Shiatsu
- Therapeutic touch
- Yoga*

*Considered in detail in later articles

Definition of complementary medicine adopted by Cochrane Collaboration

"Complementary and alternative medicine (CAM) is a broad domain of healing resources that encompasses all health systems, modalities, and practices and their accompanying theories and beliefs, other than those intrinsic to the politically dominant health system of a particular society or culture in a given historical period. CAM includes all such practices and ideas self-defined by their users as preventing or treating illness or promoting health and well-being. Boundaries within CAM and between the CAM domain and that of the dominant system are not always sharp or fixed."

Unhelpful assumptions about complementary medicine

"Non-statutory—not provided by the NHS"
- Complementary medicine is increasingly available on the NHS
- 39% of general practices provide access to complementary medicine for NHS patients

"Unregulated—therapists not regulated by state legislation"
- Osteopaths and chiropractors are now state registered and regulated, and other disciplines will probably soon follow
- Substantial amount of complementary medicine is delivered by conventional health professionals

"Unconventional—not taught in medical schools"
- Disciplines such as physiotherapy and chiropody are also not taught in medical schools
- Some medical schools have a complementary medicine component as part of the curriculum

"Natural"
- Good conventional medicine also involves rehabilitation with, say, rest, exercise, or diet
- Complementary medicine may involve unnatural practices such as injecting mistletoe or inserting needles into the skin

"Holistic—treats the whole person"
- Many conventional healthcare professionals work in a holistic manner
- Complementary therapists can be narrow and reductionist in their approach
- Holism relates more to outlook of practitioner than to the type of medicine practised

"Alternative"
- Implies use instead of conventional treatment
- Most users of complementary medicine seem not to have abandoned conventional medicine

"Unproved"
- There is a growing body of evidence that certain complementary therapies are effective in certain clinical conditions
- Many conventional healthcare practices are not supported by the results of controlled clinical trials

"Irrational—no scientific basis"
- Scientific research is starting to uncover the mechanisms of some complementary therapies, such as acupuncture and hypnosis

"Harmless"
- There are reports of serious adverse effects associated with using complementary medicine

Organisational structure

Historical development

Since the inception of the NHS, the public sector has supported training, regulation, research, and practice in conventional health care. The recent development of complementary medicine has taken place largely in the private sector. Until recently, most complementary practitioners trained in small, privately funded colleges and then worked independently in relative isolation from other practitioners.

Research

More complementary medical research exists than is commonly recognised—the *Cochrane Library* lists over 4000 randomised trials—but the field is still poorly researched compared with conventional medicine. There are several reasons for this, some of which also apply to conventional disciplines like occupational and speech therapy. However, complementary practitioners are increasingly aware of the value of research, and many complementary training courses now include research skills. Conventional sources of funding, such as the NHS research and development programme and major cancer charities, have become more open to complementary researchers.

Training

Although complementary practitioners (other than osteopaths and chiropractors) can legally practise without any training whatsoever, most have completed some further education in their chosen discipline.

There is great variation in the many training institutions. For the major therapies—osteopathy, chiropractic, acupuncture, herbal medicine, and homoeopathy—these tend to be highly developed, some with university affiliation, degree level exams, and external assessment. Others, particularly those teaching less invasive therapies such as reflexology and aromatherapy, tend to be small and isolated, determine curricula internally, and have idiosyncratic assessment procedures. In some courses direct clinical contact is limited. Some are not recognised by the main registering bodies in the relevant discipline. Most complementary practitioners finance their training without state support, and many train part time over several years.

Conventional healthcare practitioners such as nurses and doctors often have their own separate training courses in complementary medicine.

Regulation

Apart from osteopaths and chiropractors, complementary practitioners are not obliged to join any official register before setting up in practice. However, many practitioners are now members of appropriate registering or accrediting bodies. There are between 150 and 300 such organisations, with varying membership size and professional standards. Some complementary disciplines have as many as 50 registering organisations, all with different criteria and standards.

Recognising that this situation is unsatisfactory, many disciplines are taking steps to become unified under one regulatory body per discipline. Such bodies should, as a minimum, have published criteria for entry, established codes of conduct, complaints procedures, and disciplinary sanctions and should require members to be fully insured.

The General Osteopathic Council and General Chiropractic Council have been established by acts of parliament and have statutory self regulatory status and similar powers and functions to those of the General Medical Council. A small number of other disciplines—such as acupuncture, herbal medicine, and homoeopathy—have a single main regulatory body and are working towards statutory self regulation.

Factors limiting research in complementary medicine

Lack of funding—In 1995 only 0.08% of NHS research funds were spent on complementary medicine. Many funding bodies have been reluctant to give grants for research in complementary medicine. Pharmaceutical companies have little commercial interest in researching complementary medicine

Lack of research skills—Complementary practitioners usually have no training in critical evaluation of existing research or practical research skills

Lack of an academic infrastructure—This means limited access to computer and library facilities, statistical support, academic supervision, and university research grants

Insufficient patient numbers—Individual list sizes are small, and most practitioners have no disease "specialty" and therefore see very small numbers of patients with the same clinical condition. Recruiting patients into studies is difficult in private practice

Difficulty undertaking and interpreting systematic reviews—Many poor quality studies make interpretation of results difficult. Many publications in complementary medicine are not on standard databases such as Medline. Many different types of treatment exist within each complementary discipline (for example, formula, individualised, electro, laser, and auricular acupuncture)

Methodological issues—Responses to treatment are unpredictable and individual, and treatment is usually not standardised. Designing appropriate controls for some complementary therapies (such as acupuncture, manipulation) is difficult, as is blinding patients to treatment allocation. Allowing for the role of the therapeutic relationship also creates problems

---

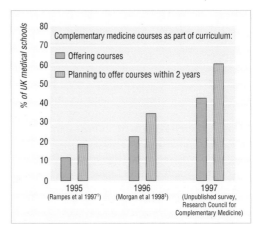

Numbers of medical schools offering or planning to offer courses on complementary medicine as part of the curriculum

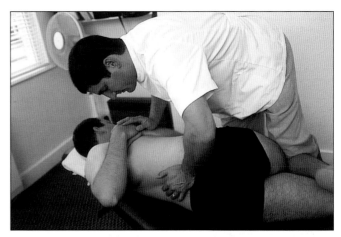

The General Osteopathic Council and General Chiropractic Council have been established by acts of parliament to regulate their respective disciplines

Efficient regulation of the "less invasive" complementary therapies such as massage or relaxation therapies is equally important. However, statutory regulation, with its requirements for parliamentary legislation and expensive bureaucratic procedures, may not be feasible. Legal and ethics experts argue that unified and efficient voluntary self regulatory bodies that fulfil the minimum standards listed above should be sufficient to safeguard patients. It will be some years before even this is achieved across the board.

Approaches to treatment

The approaches used by different complementary practitioners have some common features. Although they are not shared by all complementary disciplines, and some apply to conventional disciplines as well, understanding them may help to make sense of patients' experiences of complementary medicine.

The holistic approach

Many, but not all, complementary practitioners have a multifactorial and multilevel view of human illness. Disease is thought to result from disturbances at a combination of physical, psychological, social, and spiritual levels. The body's capacity for self repair, given appropriate conditions, is emphasised.

According to most complementary practitioners, the purpose of therapeutic intervention is to restore balance and facilitate the body's own healing responses rather than to target individual disease processes or stop troublesome symptoms. They may therefore prescribe a package of care, which could include modification of lifestyle, dietary change, and exercise as well as a specific treatment. Thus, a medical herbalist may give counselling, an exercise regimen, guidance on breathing and relaxation, dietary advice, and a herbal prescription.

It should be stressed that this holistic approach is not unique to complementary practice. Good conventional general practice, for example, follows similar principles.

Use of unfamiliar terms and ideas

Complementary practitioners often use terms and ideas that are not easily translated into Western scientific language. For example, neither the reflex zones manipulated in reflexology nor the "Qi energy" fundamental to traditional Chinese medicine have any known anatomical or physiological correlates.

Sometimes familiar terms are used but with a different meaning: acupuncturists may talk of "taking the pulse," but they will be assessing characteristics such as "wiriness" or "slipperiness," which have no Western equivalent. It is important not to interpret terms used in complementary medicine too literally and to understand that they are sometimes used metaphorically or as a shorthand for signs, symptoms, and syndromes that are not recognised in conventional medicine.

Different categorisation of illness

Complementary and conventional practitioners often have very different methods of assessing and diagnosing patients. Thus, a patient's condition may be described as "deficient liver Qi" by a traditional acupuncturist, a "pulsatilla constitution" by a homoeopath, and "a peptic ulcer" by a conventional doctor. In each case the way the problem is diagnosed determines the treatment given.

Confusingly, there is little correlation between the different diagnostic systems: some patients with deficient liver Qi do not have ulcers, and some ulcer patients do not have deficient liver

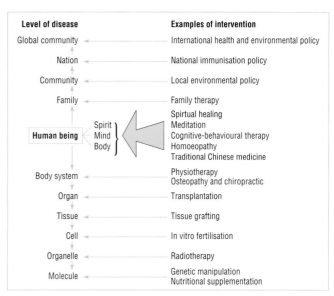

There are multiple levels of disease and, therefore, multiple levels at which therapeutic interventions can be made

Example of a holistic approach—Rudolph Steiner's central tenets of anthroposophy

- Each individual is unique
- Scientific, artistic, and spiritual insights may need to be applied together to restore health
- Life has meaning and purpose—the loss of this sense may lead to a deterioration in health
- Illness may provide opportunities for positive change and a new balance in our lives

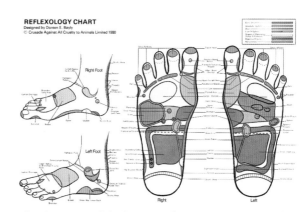

In reflexology areas of the foot are believed to correspond to the organs or structures of the body

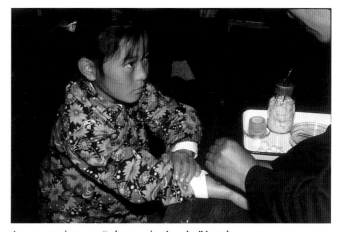

Acupuncturists may "take a patient's pulse," but they assess characteristics such as "wiriness" or "slipperiness"

Qi but another traditional Chinese diagnosis. This causes problems when comparing complementary and conventional treatments in defined patient groups.

It should be stressed that the lack of a shared world view is not necessarily a barrier to effective cooperation. For example, doctors work closely alongside hospital chaplains and social workers, each regarding the others as valued members of the healthcare team.

Approaches to learning and teaching

Complementary practitioners are not generally concerned with understanding the basic scientific mechanism of their particular therapy. Their knowledge base is often derived from a tradition of clinical observation and treatment decisions are usually empirical. Sometimes traditional teachings are handed down in a way that discourages questioning and evolution of practice, or encourages reliance on their own and others' individual anecdotal clinical and intuitive experience.

Conclusion

It is obvious from this discussion that complementary medicine is a heterogeneous subject. It is unlikely that all complementary disciplines will have an equal impact on UK health practices. The individual complementary therapies with the most immediate relevance to the medical profession are reviewed in detail in later articles, but some disciplines are inevitably beyond the scope of this series—most notably those related to healing—and interested readers should consult texts listed in the boxes.

The ABC of complementary medicine is edited and written by Catherine Zollman and Andrew Vickers. Catherine Zollman is a general practitioner in Bristol, and Andrew Vickers will shortly take up a post at Memorial Sloan-Kettering Cancer Center, New York. At the time of writing, both worked for the Research Council for Complementary Medicine, London. The series will be published as a book in Spring 2000.

1 Rampes H, Sharples F, Maragh S, Fisher P. Introducing complementary medicine into the medical curriculum. *J R Soc Med* 1997;90:19-22.
2 Morgan D, Glanville H, Mars S, Nathanson V. Education and training in complementary and alternative medicine: a postal survey of UK universities, medical schools and faculties of nurse education. *Complementary Ther Med* 1998;6: 64-70.

Sources of information on healing

National Federation of Spiritual Healers (NFSH)
Largest professional registering body
Old Manor Farm Studio, Church Street, Sunbury on Thames, Middlesex TW16 6RG. Tel: 01932 783164. Fax: 01932 779648.
URL: www.nfsh.org.uk

Confederation of Healing Organisations (CHO)
Umbrella organisation for registering bodies in healing
Suite J, Second Floor, The Red and White House, 113 High Street, Berkhamsted HP4 2DJ. Tel: 01442 870660

Publications
- Benor D. *Healing research.* Vols 1-4. Deddington: Helix Editions, 1992
  Review of collected research on healing
- Brown C. *Optimum healing.* London: Rider, 1998
  Description of a general practitioner's experience and use of healing

---

Further reading
- Ernst E. *Complementary medicine: a critical appraisal.* Oxford: Butterworth-Heinemann, 1996
- Lewith G, Kenyon J, Lewis P. *Complementary medicine: an integrated approach.* Oxford: Oxford University Press, 1996 (Oxford General Practice Series)
- Vickers AJ, ed. *Examining complementary medicine.* Cheltenham: Stanley Thornes, 1998
- Vincent C, Furnham A. *Complementary medicine: a research perspective.* London: Wiley, 1997
- Woodham A, Peters D. *An encyclopaedia of complementary medicine.* London: Dorling Kindersley, 1997

---

2 Users and practitioners of complementary medicine

Complementary medicine seems to be becoming more popular in Britain. Media coverage, specialist publications, and numbers of complementary therapists have all increased dramatically in the past 20 years. In this chapter we analyse this phenomenon and review available evidence about the use of complementary medicine.

Surveys of use

Several surveys, of varying quality, have been undertaken, but interpretation is not straightforward. Some studies targeted practitioners, whereas others surveyed patients and consumers. Different definitions of complementary medicine have been used—some include only patients consulting one of five named types of complementary practitioner, while some include up to 14 different therapies and others include complementary medicines bought over the counter. When treatments such as hypnosis are given by conventional doctors or within conventional health services, patients and surveys may not register them as "complementary." However, it is possible to make estimates from the available data, which help to chart the development of complementary practice.

Levels of use

How many people use complementary medicine?
The most rigorous UK survey of use of complementary medicine estimated that, in 1993, 33% of the population had used some form of complementary medicine and that over 10% had consulted a complementary practitioner in the previous year. Surveys of patients with chronic and difficult to manage diseases—such as cancer, HIV infection, multiple sclerosis, psoriasis, and rheumatological conditions—give levels of use up to twice as high.

Comparisons can be made with figures from other countries, although variations may be partly due to differences in survey methodology.

How extensively is complementary medicine used?
Attempts have been made to estimate the number of complementary medicine consultations taking place in the United Kingdom. In 1993 there were about 12 million adult consultations in the six major complementary disciplines. Average consultation rates were 4.3 per patient. Estimates based on the increased number of registered complementary practitioners suggest that at least 15 million complementary medicine consultations took place in 1997, about 5% of the number of general practice consultations.

Which therapies are used?
The media often emphasise the more unusual and controversial therapies, but surveys show that most use of complementary therapy is confined to a few major disciplines. Osteopathy, chiropractic, homoeopathy, acupuncture, and herbalism are among the most popular in the United Kingdom. Spiritual healing and hypnotherapy are also often mentioned. These figures mask variations in the use of individual complementary therapies among various subsections of the population. For example, although women use more complementary medicine

Use of complementary medicine in UK surveys

Survey	% of sample using complementary medicine		No of types of therapy surveyed
	Ever used	In past year	
Research Surveys of Great Britain (RSGB) 1984	30%*	No data	14
Gallup 1986	14%	No data	6
Which? 1986	No data	14%	5
MORI 1989	27%*	No data	13
Thomas 1993†	16.9% (33%*)	10.5%	6‡

Data from Sharma 1995 and Research Council for Complementary Medicine 1998. *Includes over the counter medicines. †Most rigorous study to date. ‡Plus "Other CM practitioner."

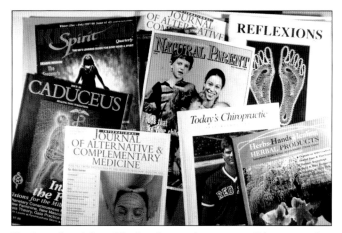

Numbers of specialist publications for complementary medicine are growing

Use of complementary medicine worldwide

Country	% of sample using complementary medicine	
	Seeing a practitioner	Using any form of treatment
United Kingdom	10.5% in past year	33% ever
Australia	20% in past year	46% in past year
United States	11% in past year	34% in past year
Belgium	24% in past year	66-75% ever
France	No data	49% ever
Netherlands	6-7% in past year	18% ever
West Germany	5-12% in past year	20-30% ever

Data from surveys during 1987-96.

Most popular complementary disciplines in UK surveys

Top five therapies in survey			
RSGB 1984	Which? 1986	MORI 1989*†	Thomas 1993†
Acupuncture	Acupuncture	Acupuncture	Acupuncture
Chiropractic	Chiropractic	Chiropractic	Chiropractic
Herbal medicine‡	Herbalism	Faith healing	Herbalism
Homoeopathy	Homoeopathy	Homoeopathy	Homoeopathy
Osteopathy	Osteopathy	Osteopathy	Osteopathy

Data from Sharma 1995 and Research Council for Complementary Medicine 1998. *Did not include herbalism. †Asked about consultations with complementary practitioners only. ‡Included over the counter products.

overall, men are more likely to consult osteopaths and chiropractors.

The popularity of different complementary therapies varies considerably across Europe. This reflects differences in medical culture and in the historical, political, and legal position of complementary medicine in these countries.

Reasons for use

There are many myths and stereotypes about people who turn to complementary medicine—for example, that they have an alternative world view which rejects conventional medicine on principle or that they are lured by exaggerated advertising claims. The research evidence challenges such theories.

Qualitative and quantitative studies show that people who consult complementary practitioners usually have longstanding conditions for which conventional medicine has not provided a satisfactory solution, either because it is insufficiently effective or because it causes adverse effects. They have generally already consulted a conventional healthcare practitioner for the problem, and many continue to use the two systems concurrently. Some "pick and mix" between complementary and conventional care, claiming that there are certain problems for which their general practitioner has the best approach and others for which a complementary practitioner is more appropriate. Most find their complementary practitioners through personal recommendation.

Once complementary therapy is started, patients' ongoing use can be broadly classified into four categories—earnest seekers, stable users, eclectic users, and one-off users. Decisions about using complementary medicine are often complex and reflect different and overlapping concerns. It is too early to assess whether the increasing availability of complementary medicine on the NHS is changing either the types of people who use complementary medicine or their reasons for doing so.

Who uses complementary medicine?
Survey data give us some idea of the characteristics of complementary medicine users in the United Kingdom.
● About 55-65% of those who consult complementary practitioners are female, a similar proportion to users of conventional healthcare
● The highest users are those aged 35-60 (users of conventional healthcare services tend to be the very old and the very young)
● Children make up a relatively small proportion of users of complementary medicine, but individual therapies differ: nearly a third of the patients of some homoeopaths are aged under 14, whereas acupuncturists, herbalists, and chiropractors see comparatively few children
● Users of complementary medicine tend to be in higher socioeconomic groups and have higher levels of education than users of conventional care
● There has been little research into ethnicity and use of complementary medicine in Britain
● More people use complementary medicine in the south of England than in Wales, Scotland, and the north of England, but evidence suggests that this reflects access to and availability of complementary practitioners rather than any fundamental regional differences in public attitudes or interest.

Are users psychologically distinct?
Some surveys have found greater psychological morbidity, and more scepticism and negative experiences with conventional medicine, among users of complementary medicine compared with users of conventional medicine. These are not necessarily inherent differences and probably reflect the fact that most

Popularity of different complementary therapies among users in Europe

	% of sample using each therapy			
	Belgium	Denmark	France	Netherlands
Acupuncture	19	12	21	16
Homoeopathy	56	28	32	31
Manipulation	19	23	7	No data
Herbalism	31	No data	12	No data
Reflexology	No data	39	No data	No data

Data from Fisher 1994

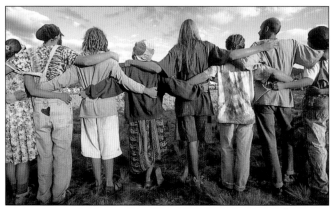

Stereotypes about use of complementary medicine being associated with alternative lifestyles are not supported by the research evidence

Recognised patterns of use of complementary medicine*
Earnest seekers—Have an intractable health problem for which they try many different forms of treatment
Stable users—Either use one type of therapy for most of their healthcare problems or have one main problem for which they use a regular package of one or more complementary therapies
Eclectic users—Choose and use different forms of therapy depending on individual problems and circumstances
One-off users—Discontinue complementary treatment after limited experimentation

*Modified from Sharma 1995

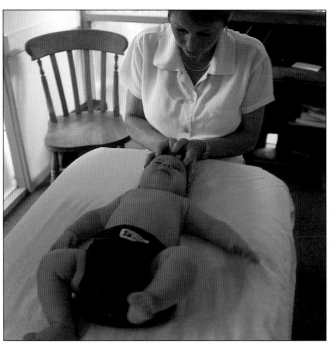

Child receiving cranial osteopathy

people who turn to complementary medicine do so for difficult, persisting problems that have not responded to conventional treatments.

Some heterogeneity between users of different therapies has been identified—for example, acupuncture patients tend to have the most chronic medical history and to be the least satisfied with their conventional treatment and general practitioner.

What conditions are treated?

Over three quarters of patients presenting to practitioners of the major complementary disciplines have a musculoskeletal problem as their main complaint. Neurological, psychological, and allergic disorders are also common. Others have problems that are not easy to categorise conventionally, such as lack of energy, and some have no specific problems but want to maintain a level of general "wellness." Case mix varies by therapy: for example, homoeopaths and herbalists tend to treat conditions such as eczema, menstrual problems, and headaches more often than musculoskeletal problems.

Complementary practitioners

The number and profile of complementary practitioners is changing rapidly. In 1981 about 13 500 registered practitioners were working in the United Kingdom. By 1997 this figure had trebled to about 40 000, with three disciplines—healing, aromatherapy, and reflexology—accounting for over half of all registered complementary practitioners, with roughly 14 000, 7000, and 5000 members respectively. Although membership of these disciplines is high compared with other complementary disciplines (only 1118 chiropractors and 2325 osteopaths were registered at the time), very few practise full time.

Nearly 4000 conventional healthcare professionals also practise complementary medicine and are members of their own register (such as the British Medical Acupuncture Society for doctors and dentists). Of these, nearly half practise acupuncture (mainly doctors and physiotherapists), about a quarter practise reflexology (mainly nurses and midwives), and about one in seven practises homoeopathy (mainly doctors, chiropodists, and podiatrists). Many more conventional healthcare professionals, especially general practitioners, have attended basic training courses and provide limited forms of complementary medicine without official registration.

Complementary medicine provided by the NHS

A substantial amount of complementary medicine is provided by conventional healthcare professionals within existing NHS services, and this provision seems to be increasing. In 1987 a regional survey of general practitioners revealed that 16% practised a complementary therapy. A UK-wide survey in 1995 showed that almost 40% of all general practices offered some form of access to complementary medicine for their NHS patients, of which over 70% was paid for by the NHS. Over half of these practices provided complementary medicine via a member of the primary healthcare team, usually a general practitioner. Another local survey published in 1998 suggests that in some areas up to half of general practices provide some access to complementary medicine.

Less is known about access via secondary care, but certain specialties are more likely to provide complementary therapies. In 1998 a survey of hospices revealed that over 90% offered some complementary therapy to patients. Pain clinics, oncology units, and rehabilitation wards also often provide complementary therapies.

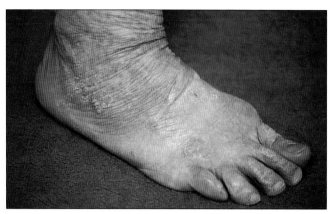

Patients are more likely to turn to complementary medicine if they have chronic, relapsing and remitting conditions such as eczema

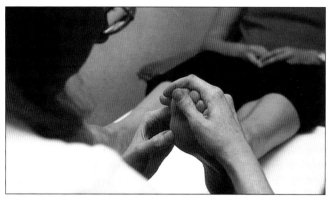

A fifth of all UK general practices provide some complementary medicine via a member of the primary healthcare team

Further reading
- Coward R. *The whole truth*. London: Faber and Faber, 1989
- Furnham A. Why do people choose and use complementary therapies? In: Ernst E, ed. *Complementary medicine, an objective appraisal*. Oxford: Butterworth Heinemann, 1998: 71-88
- Sharma U. *Complementary medicine today: practitioners and patients*. Rev ed. London: Routledge, 1995

Key references
- Mills S, Peacock W. *Professional organisation of complementary and alternative medicine in the United Kingdom 1997: a report to the Department of Health*. Exeter: Centre for Complementary Health Studies, University of Exeter, 1997
- Vickers AJ. The use of complementary therapies (letter). *BMJ* 1994;309:1161 (survey)
- Thomas K, Fall M, Parry G, Nicholl J. *National survey of access to complementary health care via general practice: report to Department of Health*. Sheffield: SCHARR, 1995
- Fisher P, Ward A. Complementary medicine in Europe. *BMJ* 1994;309:107-11
- Wearn AM, Greenfield SM. Access to complementary medicine in general practice: survey in one UK health authority. *J R Soc Med* 1998;91:465-70

The picture of "New Agers" is reproduced with permission of Morvan/Rex Features/SIPA Press. The pictures of cranial osteopathy, eczema, and reflexology are reproduced with permission of BMJ/Ulrike Preuss.

3   Complementary medicine in conventional practice

The past 10 years has seen a significant increase in the amount of complementary medicine being accessed through the NHS. These services are not evenly distributed, and many different delivery mechanisms are used, some of which (such as homoeopathic hospitals) predate the inception of the NHS. Others depend on more recent NHS reorganisations, like general practice fundholding and health commission contracting, or have been set up as evaluated pilot projects.

In general, development of these services has been demand led rather than evidence led. A few have published formal evaluations or audit reports. Some of these show benefits associated with complementary therapy—high patient satisfaction, significant improvements on validated health questionnaires compared with waiting list controls, and suggestions of reduced prescribing and referrals. However, data from other services are less clear, and many have not been formally evaluated. These pilot projects have also identified various factors that influence the integration of complementary medicine practitioners within NHS settings.

Causes for concern

While much needed evidence is gathered, the debate about more widespread integration of complementary medicine continues. The idea of providing such care within a framework of evidence based medicine, NHS reorganisations, and healthcare rationing raises various concerns for the different parties involved.

Conventional clinicians and managers want persuasive evidence that complementary medicine can deliver safe, cost effective solutions to problems that are expensive or difficult to manage with conventional treatment. Unfortunately, such evidence is both scarce and equivocal. Only a moderate number of randomised trials and very few reliable economic analyses of complementary medicine have been conducted. Moreover, no systematic process exists for collecting data on safety and adverse events.

Patients—Public surveys show that most people support increased provision of complementary medicine on the NHS, but this question is often asked in isolation and does not mean that patients would necessarily prefer complementary to conventional care. When planning services, it is essential to try to distinguish between patients' desires and defined patients' needs that can be met by complementary medicine. Patients also want to be protected from unqualified complementary practitioners and inappropriate treatments. NHS provision might go some way to ensuring certain minimum standards such as proper regulation, standardised note keeping, effective channels of communication, and participation in research. It would also facilitate ongoing medical assessment.

Complementary practitioners—Some practitioners support NHS provision because it would improve equity of access, protect their right to practise (currently vulnerable to changes in European and national legislation), and guarantee a caseload. It would also provide opportunities for inter-professional learning, career development, and research. Others fear an inevitable loss of autonomy, poorer working conditions, and domination by the medical model.

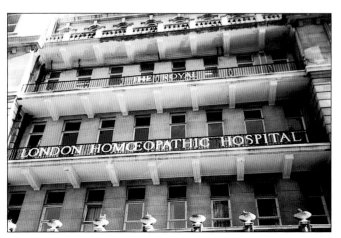

Complementary therapies have been available in the NHS since its inception

---

Integrating complementary medicine into conventional settings

Successful integration is more likely with
- Demand from patients
- Commitment from high level staff in the conventional organisation
- Protected time for education and communication
- Ongoing evaluation of service (may help to defend service in the face of financial threat)
- Links with other conventional establishments integrating complementary medicine
- Realism and good will from all parties
- Jointly agreed guidelines or protocols between complementary and conventional practitioners
- Support from senior management or health authority
- Careful selection and supervision of complementary practitioners
- Funding from charitable or voluntary sector

Problems are likely with
- Financial insecurity
- Time pressure
- Lack of appropriate premises
- Unrealistic expectations
- Overwhelming demand
- Inappropriate referrals
- Unresolved differences in perspective between complementary and conventional practitioners
- Real or perceived lack of evidence of effectiveness
- Lack of resources and time for reflection and evaluation

List adapted from the report of the Delivery Mechanisms Working Party of the Foundation for Integrated Medicine

---

Organisations promoting interdisciplinary cooperation in complementary medicine

Foundation for Integrated Medicine
Initiative of Prince of Wales, convenes working parties and events on aspects of integrated medicine
International House, 59 Compton Road, London N1 2YT. Tel: 020 7688 1881. Fax: 020 7688 1882. Email: fimed@compuserve.com

British Holistic Medical Association
Membership organisation for healthcare professionals with associate lay members
59 Lansdowne Place, Hove, East Sussex BN3 1FL. Tel/fax: 01273 725951. Email: bhma@bhma.org URL: www.bhma.org

Current provision in the NHS

In primary care

Most of the complementary medicine provided through the NHS is delivered in primary care.

Direct provision

Over 20% of primary healthcare teams provide some form complementary therapy directly. For example, general practitioners may use homoeopathy, and practice nurses may use hypnosis or reflexology. Advantages of this system are that it requires minimal financial investment and that complementary treatments are usually offered only after conventional assessment and diagnosis. Also, practitioners can monitor patients from a conventional viewpoint, ensure compliance with essential conventional medication, and identify interactions and adverse events.

A disadvantage is that shorter appointments may leave less time for non-specific aspects of the therapeutic consultation. Also, members of primary healthcare teams have often undertaken only a basic training in complementary medicine, and this generally forms only a small part of their work. Doubts about the effectiveness of the complementary treatments they deliver, compared with those given by full time complementary therapists, have been expressed. Although no comparative evidence is available, it is clear that limits of competence need to be recognised.

Indirect provision

Complementary practitioners without a background in conventional health care work in at least 20% of UK general practices. Osteopathy is the most commonly encountered profession. Such practitioners usually work privately, but some are employed by the practice and function as ancillary staff. An advantage for patients is that general practices usually check practitioners' references and credentials. Although some guidelines for referral may exist, levels of communication with general practitioners vary widely and true integration is rare.

In specialist provider units

Five NHS homoeopathic hospitals across the United Kingdom accept referrals from primary care under normal NHS conditions: free at the point of care. They offer a variety of complementary therapies provided by conventionally trained health professionals. They provide opportunities for large scale audit and evaluation of complementary medicine, but many services have been cut in recent years.

Some independent complementary medicine centres have contracts with local NHS purchasers. For example, Wessex Health Authority has a specific service contract with a private clinic to provide a multidisciplinary package of complementary medicine for NHS patients with chronic fatigue or hyperactivity. Some fundholding general practices have delegated patients to independent centres such as local chiropractic clinics rather than employ complementary practitioners in house.

A few health authorities have set up pilot projects for multidisciplinary complementary medicine in the community or on hospital premises. Advantages have included clear referral guidelines, evaluation, good communication with general practitioners, and supervised and accountable complementary practitioners. However, such centres are particularly vulnerable when health authorities come under financial pressure. Examples are the Liverpool Centre for Health and the former Lewisham Hospital NHS Trust Complementary Therapy Centre, which was closed when the local health authority had to reduce its overspend.

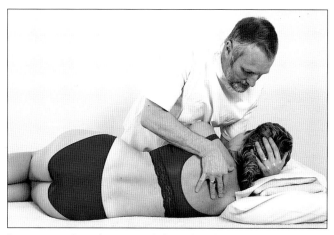

Model of provision of complementary medicine

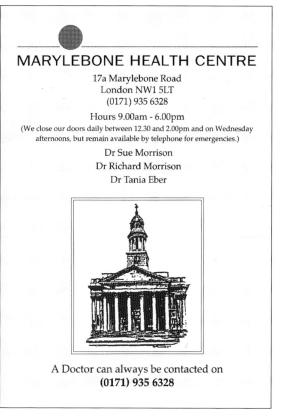

In many general practices osteopathy is provided indirectly by an independent complementary practitioner

Marylebone Health Centre was one of the first general practices to offer multidisciplinary complementary therapies to NHS patients. It provides osteopathy, massage, naturopathy, and homoeopathy

In conventional secondary care

Many NHS hospital trusts offer some form of complementary medicine to patients. This may be provided by practitioners with or without backgrounds in conventional health care. However, the availability of such services varies widely and depends heavily on local interest and high level support.

Funding for complementary medicine

Complementary medicine can be provided by conventional NHS healthcare professionals as part of everyday clinical care. This requires no special funding arrangements. General practitioners cannot claim item of service payments for complementary treatments they give to their own NHS patients.

Since 1991, health authorities can reimburse general practitioner principals who employ complementary therapists, although the staff budget is limited and a complementary practitioner is therefore employed at the expense of another member of staff. General practitioner fundholders have had additional control over staffing budgets and fundholding savings, which some have used to purchase complementary therapies. Primary care groups have greater power to allocate funds as they choose, but it remains to be seen whether complementary medicine will be identified as a priority by sufficiently large numbers of general practitioners for the creation of any new initiatives. Indeed, the change from general practice fundholding to primary care groups may mean that some established complementary services will be lost.

Local health commissions and authorities have sometimes used money for research and development, or for waiting list initiatives, to finance complementary medicine. Block service contracts or individual extracontractual referrals can be made with complementary medicine providers, but in practice financial constraints restrict this type of access.

Funds from the voluntary sector or charities may also be sought. The complementary therapy service at the Marylebone Health Centre in London was initially funded by a research grant from a charitable trust. Fundraising and donations by the local patients are now essential to its ongoing financial viability. In addition, some charities, such as the London Lighthouse for people infected with HIV, subsidise complementary medicine for people who could not otherwise afford treatment.

Some occupational health and private medical insurance schemes fund complementary therapies.

Medicolegal considerations

If doctors participate in patients' seeking complementary therapies—by advising, treating, delegating, or referring—they need to be aware of the medicolegal implications. Although each case is judged on its merits, certain guidelines apply.

Doctors who practise complementary therapies

Under the Medical Act of 1858, conventionally trained doctors can legally administer any unconventional medical treatments they choose. However, as with most medical practice, the "Bolam test" is used to determine appropriate standards of care. This means that "a doctor is not guilty of negligence if he or she has acted in accordance with a practice accepted as proper by a responsible body of medical men skilled in that particular art as long as it is subject to logical analysis." In other words, if a doctor has undergone additional training in a complementary discipline and practises in a way that is reasonable and would be considered acceptable by a number (not necessarily a majority) of other medically qualified complementary practitioners, his or her actions are defensible.

Examples of complementary medicine in secondary care	
Complementary therapy	**Healthcare professionals**
Pain clinics	
Acupuncture	Anaesthetists, physiotherapists, palliative care physicians, professional acupuncturists
Physiotherapy departments	
Manipulative therapy, acupuncture	Physiotherapists trained in manipulative medicine or acupuncture
Rheumatology departments	
Manipulative therapy	Osteopaths, chiropractors, orthopaedic physicians
Hospices	
Aromatherapy, reflexology, massage, hypnosis, relaxation, healing, acupuncture, homoeopathy	Nurses, doctors, complementary therapists, occupational therapists
Clinical psychology departments	
Hypnosis or relaxation training	Psychologists
Obstetric departments	
Yoga, acupuncture	Midwives, physiotherapists

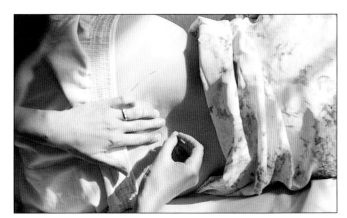

An increasing number of hospital pain clinics now offer acupuncture as a treatment for chronic pain

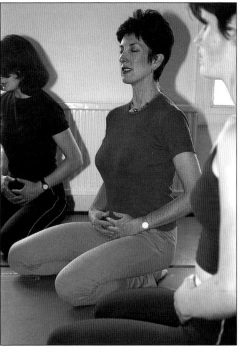

Some complementary therapies, such as relaxation, can be delivered effectively in group sessions, which improves their cost effectiveness

Referral to medically qualified practitioners
A doctor who asks another doctor to provide complementary medicine is in the same legal situation as when referring to a doctor for any other services. As long as the decision to make the referral is appropriate, all further responsibility regarding the complementary treatment is taken over by the doctor providing the specialist service.

Delegation to non-medically qualified practitioners
This situation, more than any other, concerns doctors who wish to make complementary medicine available to their patients. Despite theoretical worries, however, it is considered a very low risk area by medical defence societies. The situation may change if complementary medicine becomes more widely used.

Doctors must ask themselves three main questions:
- Is my decision to delegate to this complementary therapy appropriate?
- Have I taken reasonable steps to ensure that the practitioner concerned is qualified and insured?
- Has my medical follow up been adequate?

To date, no claims or cases have been sustained against doctors who have delegated to complementary practitioners.

Delegation to state regulated complementary practitioners
Now that osteopaths and chiropractors are state regulated, delegating to these practitioners is medicolegally similar to delegating care to a physiotherapist or other conventional healthcare professional.

Further reading
- Sharma U. *Complementary medicine today: practitioners and patients.* Rev ed. London: Routledge, 1995
- Fulder S. *The handbook of alternative and complementary medicine.* 3rd ed. Oxford: Oxford University Press, 1996
- Stone J, Matthews J. *Complementary medicine and the law.* Oxford: Oxford University Press, 1996
- Coates J, Jobst K. Integrated healthcare, a way forward for the next five years? *J Alternative Complement Med* 1998;4:209-47
- *Complementary medicine: new approaches to good practice.* Oxford: Oxford University Press, 1993

The pictures of Royal London Homoeopathic Hospital and acupuncture are reproduced with permission of the Royal London Homoeopathic Hospital. The picture of osteopathy is reproduced with permission of the General Osteopathic Council. The picture of group therapy is reproduced with permission of BMJ/Ulrike Preuss.

Medicolegally acceptable delegation to non-medically qualified complementary practitioners
Initial decision to delegate to a practitioner must pass Bolam test
- Evidence based decisions are most persuasive
- Commonly accepted but unproved indications are also acceptable

Doctors must take reasonable steps to ascertain that practitioners are appropriately qualified
- It is usually sufficient for delegating doctors to ensure that they are a member of the main professional regulatory body responsible for that particular discipline
- The main bodies require members to be fully indemnified

Doctors must retain "overall clinical responsibility"—that is, ensure appropriate follow up, reassessment, etc
- Doctors should not issue repeat complementary prescriptions without having or obtaining sufficient information to ensure safe prescribing

Obtaining lists of the main professional registers
Council for Complementary and Alternative Medicine (CCAM)
Deals with registration of acupuncture, herbal medicine, homoeopathy, and osteopathy
63 Jeddo Road, London W12 6HQ. Tel: 020 8735 0632

British Complementary Medicine Association (BCMA)
Deals with registration of wide range of complementary practitioners including reflexologists, aromatherapists, craniosacral therapists, nutritional therapists, and hypnotherapists
249 Fosse Road South, Leicester LE3 1AE. Tel: 0116 282 5511

Key evaluation reports from NHS complementary medicine services
- Richardson J. *Complementary therapy in the NHS: a service evaluation of the first year of an outpatient service in a local district general hospital.* November 1995. Report prepared by Health Services Research and Evaluation Unit, Lewisham Hospital NHS Trust, London
- Hotchkiss J. *Liverpool Centre for Health: the first year of a service offering complementary therapies on the NHS.* Liverpool: Liverpool Public Health Observatory, 1995 (Observatory Report Series No 25)
- Hills D, Welford R. *Complementary therapy in general practice: an evaluation of the Glastonbury Health Centre Complementary Medicine Service.* Somerset Trust for Integrated Health Care, 1998
- Rees R. Evaluating complementary therapy on the NHS: a critique of reports from three pilot projects. *Complement Ther Med* 1996:254-7
- Scheurmier N, Breen AC. A pilot study of the purchase of manipulation services for acute low back pain in the United Kingdom. *J Manipulative Physiol Ther* 1998;21:14-8

4 Acupuncture

Acupuncture is the stimulation of special points on the body, usually by the insertion of fine needles. Originating in the Far East about 2000 years ago, it has made various appearances in the history of European and north American medicine. William Osler, for example, used acupuncture therapeutically in the 19th century. Acupuncture's recent popularity in the West dates from the 1970s, when President Nixon visited China.

Background

In its original form acupuncture was based on the principles of traditional Chinese medicine. According to these, the workings of the human body are controlled by a vital force or energy called "Qi" (pronounced "chee"), which circulates between the organs along channels called meridians.

There are 12 main meridians, and these correspond to 12 major functions or "organs" of the body. Although they have the same names (such as liver, kidney, heart, etc), Chinese and Western concepts of the organs correlate only very loosely. Qi energy must flow in the correct strength and quality through each of these meridians and organs for health to be maintained. The acupuncture points are located along the meridians and provide one means of altering the flow of Qi.

Although the details of practice may differ between individual schools, all traditional acupuncture theory is based in the Daoist concept of yin and yang. Illness is seen in terms of excesses or deficiencies in various exogenous and endogenous pathogenic factors, and treatment is aimed at restoring balance. Traditional diagnoses are esoteric, such as "kidney-yang deficiency, water overflowing" or "damp heat in the bladder."

Many of the conventional health professionals who practise acupuncture have dispensed with such concepts. Acupuncture points are seen to correspond to physiological and anatomical features such as peripheral nerve junctions, and diagnosis is made in purely conventional terms. An important concept used by such acupuncturists is that of the "trigger point." This is an area of increased sensitivity within a muscle which is said to cause a characteristic pattern of referred pain in a related segment of the body. An example might be tender areas in the muscles of the neck and shoulder which relate to various patterns of headache.

It is often implied that a clear and firm distinction exists between traditional and Western acupuncture, but the two approaches overlap considerably. Moreover, traditional acupuncture is not a single, historically stable therapy. There are many different schools—for example, Japanese practitioners differ from their Chinese counterparts by using mainly shallow needle insertion.

Acupressure involves firm manual pressure on selected acupuncture points. Shiatsu, a modified form of acupressure, was systematised as part of traditional Japanese medicine.

How does acupuncture work?

The effects of acupuncture, particularly on pain, are at least partially explicable within a conventional physiological model. Acupuncture is known to stimulate A delta fibres entering the dorsal horn of the spinal cord. These mediate segmental inhibition of pain impulses carried in the slower, unmyelinated

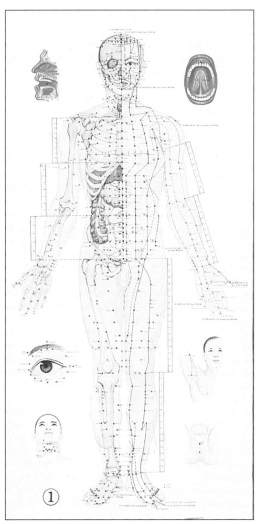

Acupuncture meridians run superficially and longitudinally. Both traditional and Western acupuncturists identify acupuncture points by their location on the meridians—for example, gall bladder 30 or large intestine 4

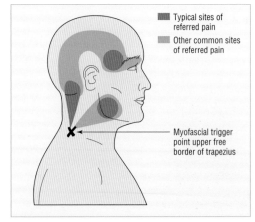

Trigger points, and their characteristic patterns of referred pain, can be treated by direct needling at the trigger point. This concept is also used in musculoskeletal medicine, with trigger points being treated by manipulative techniques

C fibres and, through connections in the midbrain, enhance descending inhibition of C fibre pain impulses at other levels of the spinal cord. This helps explain why acupuncture needles in one part of the body can affect pain sensation in another region. Acupuncture is also known to stimulate release of endogenous opioids and other neurotransmitters such as serotonin. This is likely to be another mechanism for acupuncture's effects, such as in acute pain and in substance misuse.

However, certain aspects of traditional acupuncture, which have some empirical support, resist conventional explanation. In one unreplicated study, for example, blinded assessment of the tenderness of points on the ear had high agreement with the true location of chronic pain in distant parts of the body. Changes in the electrical conductivity of acupuncture points associated with a particular organ have also been recorded in patients with corresponding conventional diseases. There are no known anatomical or physiological explanations for these observations.

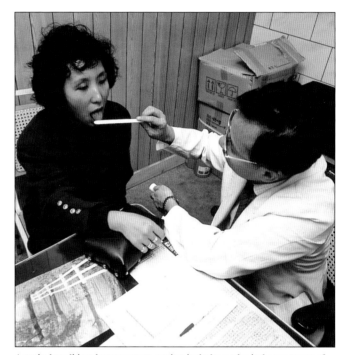

The neuronal connections which are thought to mediate the effects of acupuncture on pain

What happens during a treatment?

Traditional acupuncturists supplement a detailed, multisystem case history with observations that are said to give information about the patient's state of health. These include examination of the shape, coating, and colour of the tongue; the colour of the face; and the strength, rhythm, and quality of the pulse. Both Western and traditional practitioners may palpate to identify points at which pressure causes tenderness or pain.

Typically, between four and 10 points are needled during an acupuncture session. The needles are usually left in place for 10-30 minutes, although some practitioners needle for only a few seconds or minutes. Needles may be stimulated by manual twirling or a small electrical current. Lasers are sometimes used to stimulate acupuncture points instead of needles. Acupuncture needles are extremely fine and do not hurt in the same way as, say, an injection. Patients may even be unaware that a needle has been inserted. However, some acupuncturists attempt to produce a sensation called "de Qi"—a sense of heaviness, soreness, or numbness at the point of needling. This is said to be a sign that an acupuncture point has been correctly stimulated. Many patients say that they find acupuncture a relaxing or sedating experience.

Traditional acupuncturists may use various adjunctive therapies, including moxibustion (the burning of a herb just above the surface of the skin), massage, cupping, herbal preparations, exercises, and dietary modification.

A typical course of acupuncture treatment for a chronic condition would be six to 12 sessions over a three month period. This might be followed by "top up" treatments every two to six months.

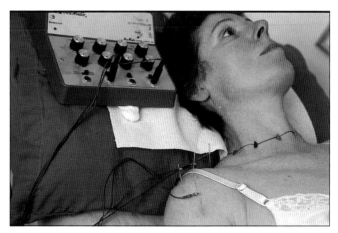

A typical traditional acupuncture session includes a physical assessment of yin-yang energy status with methods such as pulse and tongue diagnosis

Therapeutic scope

Acupuncture was developed as a relatively global system of medicine. Some current textbooks refer to treating conditions as varied as diarrhoea, the common cold, and tinnitus. As practised in Europe and north America, acupuncture is primarily a treatment for benign, chronic disease and for musculoskeletal injury. The most common presenting complaints found in surveys of acupuncture practice include back pain, arthritis, headache, asthma, hay fever, anxiety, fatigue, menstrual disorders, and digestive disorders. Acupuncture is also used in drug and alcohol rehabilitation, particularly in the United States.

Using electricity to stimulate acupuncture points is thought to augment the therapeutic effect of needling and is used particularly in treating chronic pain

Research evidence

There is good research evidence that acupuncture has effects greater than placebo. Randomised trials have found that true acupuncture is more effective in relieving pain than a "sham" technique, such as inserting needles away from true points. Of the numerous studies on nausea, a condition that readily lends itself to placebo controlled trials, almost all show that stimulating true acupuncture points is more effective that stimulating false points. Studies showing that acupuncture can affect anaesthetised animals provides further evidence that its effects probably cannot be explained purely in psychological terms.

It is less clear whether acupuncture has clinically important benefits in the conditions for which it is typically used. Much of the research evidence comes from hospital based studies of acute conditions such as postoperative pain rather than studies of chronic conditions in primary care. Moreover, most trials have had small numbers of patients and only short term follow up. Overall, evidence from several randomised controlled trials supports the use of acupuncture in pain conditions, particularly migraine, headache, and postoperative pain. Such trials also provide evidence of an effect of acupuncture in substance misuse, nausea, and stroke. Trials of acupuncture in asthma and hay fever have produced conflicting results. Systematic reviews and randomised controlled trials suggest that acupuncture is probably not of benefit for stopping smoking, tinnitus, or obesity. Data on fatigue, digestive disorders, and anxiety are insufficient.

There is little reliable information on the relative effectiveness of the various Western and traditional forms of acupuncture.

Safety of acupuncture

As with all complementary medicine, the absence of a formal system for reporting adverse effects means that acupuncture's safety is difficult to assess. However, it seems to be a relatively safe form of treatment with a low incidence of serious adverse events. An extensive worldwide literature search identified only 193 adverse events (including relatively minor events such as bruising and dizziness) over 15 years. The more serious events were usually related to poor practice—for example, cases of hepatitis B infection typically involved bad hygiene and unregistered practitioners.

A prospective study of over 55 000 acupuncture treatments given in a college for medically trained acupuncturists confirms that acupuncture is probably safe in qualified hands. Only 63, mostly minor, adverse events were identified, and no cases of serious adverse events such as pneumothorax, infection, or spinal lesions were reported, although these have been described in the literature.

Indwelling "press" needles are commonly used in the treatment of addiction and should be used with care. They have been associated with infections, such as perichondritis. Systemic infection seems to be very uncommon, but acupuncture should probably be avoided in patients with valvular heart defects. Deep needling is contraindicated in patients with bleeding disorders or taking anticoagulant drugs.

Practitioners

Acupuncturists without a background in conventional health care tend to work in private practice and treat a wide variety of conditions. About 2000 doctors and physiotherapists practise acupuncture, but they rarely specialise in it and generally use it as an adjunctive treatment when appropriate. Most offer

Key studies of efficacy

Systematic reviews
- Vickers AJ. Can acupuncture have specific effects on health? A systematic review of acupuncture antiemesis trials. *J R Soc Med* 1996;89:303-11
- White AR, Rampes H. Acupuncture for smoking cessation. In: Cochrane Collaboration. *The Cochrane Library.* Issue 2. Oxford: Update Software, 1998

Randomised controlled trials
- Johansson K, Lindgren I, Widner H, Wiklund I, Johansson BB. Can sensory stimulation improve the functional outcome in stroke patients? *Neurology* 1993;43:2189-92
- Vincent CA. A controlled trial of the treatment of migraine by acupuncture. *Clin J Pain* 1989;5:305-12

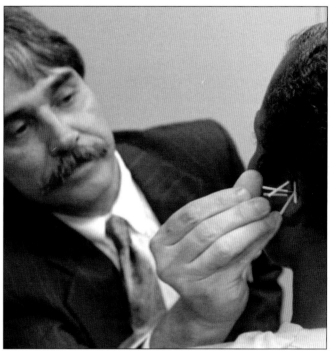

On balance, research evidence supports the use of acupuncture in treating substance misuse. Auricular acupuncture is often used for this purpose

Adverse events related to acupuncture

Reported adverse events	No of cases*
Forgotten needles (all later retrieved without sequelae)	16
Transient hypotension	13
Burn injury (such as caused by moxibustion)	6
Ecchymosis with pain	6
Ecchymosis without pain	5
Malaise	5
Minor haemorrhage	3
Aggravation of complaint	3
Suspected contact dermatitis	3
Pain in the puncture region	2
Fall from bed	1

From Yamashita H, Tsukayama H, Tanno Y, Nishijo K. Adverse events related to acupuncture [letter]. *JAMA* 1998;280:1563-4

*Total number of treatments was 55 291, from November 1992 to October 1997

treatment mainly directed at musculoskeletal and other painful conditions and are usually based in pain clinics or in general practice.

Training

Professional acupuncturists train for up to 3-4 years full time and may acquire university degrees on completion of their training. Some complete further training in the principles and practice of Chinese herbalism. All accredited acupuncture training courses include conventional anatomy, physiology, pathology, and diagnosis. Research and audit skills are also taught.

Medical acupuncturists generally have fewer training hours in acupuncture techniques—a course of several weekends in which they learn a small range of simple techniques is typical. Other conventional healthcare disciplines run courses for their own members, ranging from basic introductions to two year training in advanced acupuncture.

Regulation

Professional acupuncturists have a single regulatory body, the British Acupuncture Council (BAcC), with about 1500 members. The council aims to achieve statutory regulation, although no final decisions have been made. All members have undergone a training independently accredited by the British Acupuncture Accreditation Board. Physiotherapists are regulated by the Acupuncture Association of Chartered Physiotherapists (AACP). Although many doctors practise some basic acupuncture without an official qualification, the British Medical Acupuncture Society offers a Certificate of Basic Competence and a Diploma of Medical Acupuncture for appropriately trained doctors.

Organisations concerned with regulation and training in acupuncture

British Medical Acupuncture Society
For doctors only
Newton House, Whitley, Warrington WA4 4JA. Tel: 01925 730727. Fax: 01925 730492. Email: bmasadmin@aol.com. URL: www.medical-acupuncture.co.uk

British Acupuncture Council
63 Jeddo Road, London W12 9HQ. Tel: 020 8735 0400. Fax: 020 8735 0404. URL: www.acupuncture.org.uk

Acupuncture Association of Chartered Physiotherapists
Chartered Society of Physiotherapists, 14 Bedford Row, London WC1R 4ED. Tel: 020 7242 1941

Further reading

- Filshie J, White A. *Medical acupuncture*. Edinburgh: Churchill Livingstone, 1997
- Maciocia G. *The foundations of Chinese medicine*. Edinburgh: Churchill Livingstone, 1989
- Kaptchuk T. *Chinese medicine: the web that has no weaver*. London: Rider, 1983
- Acupuncture Resource Research Centre website. www.demon.co.uk/acupuncture/arrc.html

The chart of acupuncture points is reproduced with permission of Medicine and Health Publishing, Hong Kong, and was supplied by Scarboroughs. The diagrams showing trigger points and neuronal connections mediating acupuncture's effects were supplied by Mike Cummings of the British Medical Acupuncture Society. The picture of tongue examination is reproduced with permission of Mark de Fraye/ Science Photo Library. The picture of auricular acupuncture is reproduced with permission of AP/Shane Young. The picture of electrically stimulated acupuncture is reproduced with permission of BMJ/Ulrike Preuss.

5 Herbal medicine

Background

The use of plants for healing purposes predates human history and forms the origin of much modern medicine. Many conventional drugs originate from plant sources: a century ago, most of the few effective drugs were plant based. Examples include aspirin (from willow bark), digoxin (from foxglove), quinine (from cinchona bark), and morphine (from the opium poppy). The development of drugs from plants continues, with drug companies engaged in large scale pharmacological screening of herbs.

Chinese herbalism is the most prevalent of the ancient herbal traditions currently practised in Britain. It is based on concepts of yin and yang and of Qi energy. Chinese herbs are ascribed qualities such as "cooling" (yin) or "stimulating" (yang) and used, often in combination, according to the deficiencies or excesses of these qualities in the patient.

Modern Western herbalism emphasises the effects of herbs on individual body systems. For example, herbs may be used for their supposed anti-inflammatory, haemostatic, expectorant, antispasmodic, or immunostimulatory properties.

Spending on herbal products in the United Kingdom is over £40m a year, mainly from self prescription of over the counter products. This type of herbal drug use is typically based on a simple matching of a particular herb to particular diseases or symptoms—such as valerian (*Valeriana officinalis*) for sleep disturbance. Originally confined to health food shops, herbal remedies are now marketed in many conventional pharmacies.

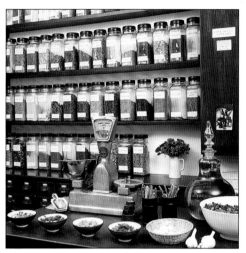

Until a century ago most effective medicines were plant based

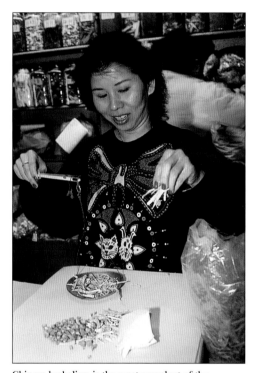

Chinese herbalism is the most prevalent of the traditional herbal practices in Britain

Differences from conventional drug use

Although superficially similar, herbal medicine and conventional pharmacotherapy have three important differences:

Use of whole plants—Herbalists generally use unpurified plant extracts containing several different constituents. They claim that these can work together synergistically so that the effect of the whole herb is greater than the summed effects of its components. They also claim that toxicity is reduced when whole herbs are used instead of isolated active ingredients ("buffering"). Although two samples of a particular herbal drug may contain constituent compounds in different proportions, practitioners claim that this does not generally cause clinical problems. There is some experimental evidence for synergy and buffering in certain whole plant preparations, but how far this is generalisable to all herbal products is not known.

Herb combining—Often, several different herbs are used together. Practitioners say that the principles of synergy and buffering apply to combinations of plants and claim that combining herbs improves efficacy and reduces adverse effects. This contrasts with conventional practice, where polypharmacy is generally avoided whenever possible.

Diagnosis—Herbal practitioners use different diagnostic principles from conventional practitioners. For example, when treating arthritis, they might observe "underfunctioning of a patient's systems of elimination" and decide that the arthritis results from "an accumulation of metabolic waste products." A diuretic, choleretic, or laxative combination of herbs might then be prescribed alongside herbs with anti-inflammatory properties.

Example of a herbal prescription for osteoarthritis

- Turmeric (*Curcuma longa*) tincture 20 ml—For anti-inflammatory activity and to improve local circulation at affected joints
- Devil's claw (*Harpagophytum procumbens*) tincture 30 ml—For anti-inflammatory activity and general wellbeing
- Ginseng (*Panax* spp) tincture 10 ml—For weakness and exhaustion
- White willow (*Salix alba*) tincture 20 ml—For anti-inflammatory activity
- Liquorice (*Glycyrrhiza glabra*) 5 ml—For anti-inflammatory activity and to improve palatability and absorption of herbal medicine
- Oats (*Avena sativa*) 15 ml—To aid sleep and for general wellbeing

---

What happens during a treatment?

Herbal practitioners take extensive case histories and perform a physical examination. Patients are asked to describe their medical history and current symptoms. Particular attention is paid to the state of everyday processes such as appetite, digestion, urination, defecation, and sleep. Patients are then prescribed individualised combinations of herbs. These are usually taken as tinctures (alcoholic extracts) or teas. Syrups, pills, capsules, ointments, and compresses may also be used. Oral preparations can taste and smell unpleasant.

In addition to the herbal prescription, practitioners may work with their clients to improve diet and other lifestyle factors such as exercise and emotional issues. Follow up appointments occur after two to four weeks. Progress is reviewed and changes made to drugs, doses, or regimen as necessary.

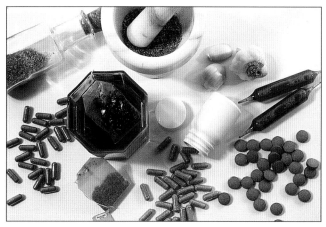

Herbal remedies are available in a wide variety of formulations

Therapeutic scope

Although herbal preparations are widely used as self medication for acute conditions, practitioners of herbal medicine tend to concentrate on treating chronic conditions. A typical caseload might include asthma, eczema, premenstrual syndrome, rheumatoid arthritis, migraine, menopausal symptoms, chronic fatigue, and irritable bowel syndrome. Herbalists do not tend to treat acute mental or musculoskeletal disorders.

The aim of herbal treatment is usually to produce persisting improvements in wellbeing. Practitioners often talk in terms of trying to treat the "underlying cause" of disease and may prescribe herbs aimed at correcting patterns of dysfunction rather than targeting the presenting symptoms. That said, many practitioners prescribe symptomatically as well, such as giving a remedy to aid sleep in a patient with chronic pain.

Research evidence

In laboratory settings plant extracts have been shown to have a variety of pharmacological effects, including anti-inflammatory, vasodilatory, antimicrobial, anticonvulsant, sedative, and antipyretic effects. In a typical study an infusion of lemon grass leaves produced a dose dependent reduction of experimentally induced hyperalgesia in rat.

Human studies also confirm specific therapeutic effects of particular herbs: randomised controlled trials support the use of ginger for treating nausea and vomiting, feverfew for migraine prophylaxis, and ginkgo for cerebral insufficiency and dementia. The best known evidence about a herbal product concerns St John's wort (*Hypericum perforatum*) for treating mild to moderate depression. A systematic review of 23 randomised controlled trials found the herb to be significantly superior to placebo and therapeutically equivalent to, but with fewer side effects than, antidepressants such as amitriptyline.

However, there is still very little evidence on the effectiveness of herbalism as practised—that is, using principles such as combining herbs and unconventional diagnosis. Almost no randomised studies have investigated herbal practitioners treating as they would in everyday clinical work. Perhaps the closest attempt evaluated a traditional Chinese herbal treatment of eczema. As prescriptions depend on patients' exact presentations, only those with widespread, non-exudative eczema were included. Eighty seven adults and children, refractory to conventional first and second line treatment, were randomised to a crossover study that compared a preparation of about 10 Chinese herbs with a placebo consisting of herbs thought to be ineffective for eczema. Highly significant reductions in eczema scores were associated with active

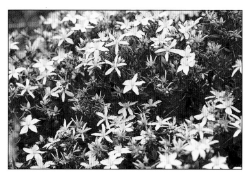

A substantial evidence base supports the use of St John's wort for treating mild to moderate depression

---

Key studies of efficacy

Systematic reviews
- Linde K, Ramirez G, Mulrow CD, Pauls A, Weidenhammer W. St John's wort for depression—an overview and meta-analysis of randomised clinical trials. *BMJ* 1996;313:253-8
- Melchart D, Linde K, Fischer P, Kaesmayr J. Echinacea for preventing and treating the common cold. In: Cochrane Collaboration. *The Cochrane Library*. Issue 3. Oxford: Update Software, 1999
- Wilt TJ, Ishani A, Stark G, MacDonald R, Lau J, Mulrow C. Saw palmetto extracts for treatment of benign prostatic hyperplasia: a systematic review. *JAMA* 1998;280:1604-9

Randomised controlled trials
- Sheehan MP, Rustin MH, Atherton DJ, Buckley C, Harris DW, Brostoff J, et al. Efficacy of traditional Chinese herbal therapy in adult atopic dermatitis. *Lancet* 1992;340:13-7

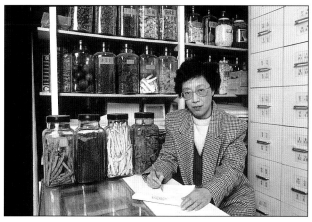

The dramatic responses of some patients' eczema after treatment by Dr Luo at the Hong Ning Co, London clinic, prompted dermatologists to undertake randomised controlled trials of the herbal treatment

treatment but not with placebo. At long term follow up, over half of the adults (12/21) and over 75% of the children (18/23) who continued treatment had a greater than 90% reduction in eczema scores.

Safety

Many plants are highly toxic. Herbal medicine probably presents a greater risk of adverse effects and interactions than any other complementary therapy. There are case reports of serious adverse events after administration of herbal products. In most cases the herbs involved were self prescribed and bought over the counter or obtained from a source other than a registered practitioner. In the most notorious instance, several women developed rapidly progressive interstitial renal fibrosis after taking Chinese herbs prescribed by a slimming clinic.

As well as their direct pharmacological effects, herbal products may be contaminated, adulterated, or misidentified. Adverse effects seem more common with herbs imported from outside Europe and north America. In general, patients taking herbal preparations regularly should receive careful follow up and have access to appropriate biochemical monitoring.

As with many complementary therapies, information on the prevalence of adverse effects is limited. The National Institute of Medical Herbalists and the University of Exeter have begun to operate a type of "yellow card" system to collect and collate adverse events reported by herbalists. The National Poisons Unit has set up a database to record adverse events and interactions, but, without a more systematic reporting scheme, the incidence of such events will remain unknown.

Interactions of herbal products with conventional drugs have been described. Some well characterised interactions exist, and competent medical herbalists are trained to take a detailed drug history and avoid these. Other interactions are not clearly defined. Problems are more likely to occur with less well qualified practitioners, more unusual combinations of agents, patients taking several conventional drugs, and those who self prescribe herbal medicines. If patients are taking conventional drugs, herbal preparations should be used with extreme caution and only on the advice of a herbalist familiar with the relevant conventional pharmacology.

Sources of information on safety of herbal products

EXTRACT database
Centre for Complementary Health Studies, Exeter University, Exeter EX4 4RG. Tel: 01392 264496

PhytoNet Home Page www.exeter.ac.uk/phytonet/
An information resource concerning development, manufacture, regulation, and surveillance of herbal medicines

National poisons units
Contact details for poisons information centres available in the *British National Formulary*

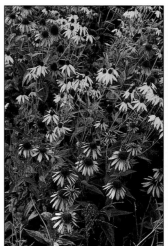 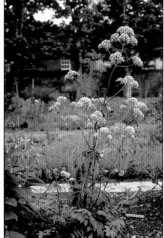

Several herbal products interact with conventional drugs—such as echinacea (left) with anabolic steroids and valerian (right) with barbiturates

Important potential interactions between herbal preparations and conventional drugs

Herb	Conventional drug	Potential problem
Echinacea used for >8 weeks	Anabolic steroids, methotrexate, amiodarone, ketoconazole	Hepatotoxicity
Feverfew	Non-steroidal anti-inflammatory drugs	Inhibition of herbal effect
Feverfew, garlic, ginseng, gingko, ginger	Warfarin	Altered prothrombin time/INR/
Ginseng	Phenelzine sulphate	Headache, tremulousness, manic episodes
Ginseng	Oestrogens, corticosteroids	Additive effects
St John's wort	Monoamine oxidase inhibitor and serotonin reuptake inhibitor antidepressants	Mechanism of herbal effect uncertain. Insufficient evidence of safety with concomitant use—therefore not advised
Valerian	Barbiturates	Additive effects, excessive sedation
Kyushin, liquorice, plantain, uzara root, hawthorn, ginseng	Digoxin	Interference with pharmacodynamics and drug level monitoring
Evening primrose oil, borage	Anticonvulsants	Lowered seizure threshold
Shankapulshpi (Ayurvedic preparation)	Phenytoin	Reduced drug levels, inhibition of drug effect
Kava	Benzodiazepines	Additive sedative effects, coma
Echinacea, zinc (immunostimulants)	Immunosuppressants (such as corticosteroids, cyclosporin)	Antagonistic effects
St John's wort, saw palmetto	Iron	Tannic acid content of herbs may limit iron absorption
Kelp	Thyroxine	Iodine content of herb may interfere with thyroid replacement
Liquorice	Spironolactone	Antagonism of diuretic effect
Karela, ginseng	Insulin, sulphonylureas, biguanides	Altered glucose concentrations. These herbs should not be prescribed in diabetic patients

Data from: Miller LG. Herbal medicinals: selected clinical considerations focusing on known or potential drug-herb interactions. *Arch Intern Med* 1998;158:2200-11

Practitioners

Herbalists generally work as sole practitioners or in complementary medicine clinics. Few have conventional healthcare qualifications. There seems to have been little penetration of herbal medicine into the NHS. A small number of doctors practise herbalism, but this is often not integrated into their NHS work. Some ethnic groups have their own indigenous herbal practitioners, such as Hakims or Ayurvedic practitioners from the Indian subcontinent.

Training

There are many different courses in herbalism and substantial variation in the content and standard of teaching. The most comprehensively trained practitioners are known as medical herbalists and are members of the National Institute of Medical Herbalists (NIMH). Their training usually includes at least 500 hours of supervised clinical practice and training in nutrition, communication skills, pharmacology, pharmacognosy, botany, pathology, conventional clinical diagnosis, biochemistry, physiology, and research skills. Courses last the equivalent of four years full time and lead to BSc degrees in herbal medicine.

Training in Chinese herbalism may be additional to a training in acupuncture or may stand on its own. Some British courses involve student placement in China.

Courses in herbal medicine for doctors range from two day introductions to two year programmes leading to a diploma in herbal medicine.

Regulation

The National Institute of Medical Herbalists was set up in 1864 and remains the main registering and regulating body for Western herbal practitioners. Only graduates of approved courses are accepted on to the register, and a strict code of ethics is maintained.

The Register of Chinese Herbal Practitioners accepts graduates from four main British colleges of Chinese herbal medicine. There is no generally accepted British register for practitioners who qualified in China.

The European Herbal Practitioners Association, an umbrella body with about 1000 members, has been set up to encourage greater unity among herbalists. However, it has no formal criteria for screening membership and no published code of ethics as yet.

Further reading

- Mills S. *The essential book of herbal medicine.* London: Arkana, 1993.
- Newall CA, Anderson LA, Phillipson JD. *Herbal medicines. a guide for health-care professionals.* London: Pharmaceutical Press, 1996

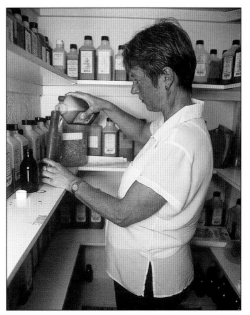

Many herbal prescriptions are individually formulated and dispensed by herbal practitioners themselves

---

Main regulatory and registering bodies in herbal medicine

National Institute of Medical Herbalists (NIMH)
56 Longbrook Street, Exeter EX4 6AH. Tel: 01392 426022.
    Fax: 01392 498963. Email: nimh@ukexeter.freeserve.co.uk
    URL: www.btinternet.com/~nimh/

Register of Chinese Herbal Medicine
PO Box 400, Wembley, Middlesex HA9 9NZ. Tel: 020 7470 8740
    URL: www.rchm.co.uk

European Herbal Practitioners Association
Midsummer Cottage Clinic, Nether Westcote, Chipping Norton OX7 6SD. Tel: 01993 830419. Fax: 01993 830957
    URL: www.users.globalnet.co.uk/~epha/

The picture of a herbal dispensary is reproduced with permission of Paul Biddle/Science Photo Library. The pictures of Chinese herbal medicine are reproduced with permission of Rex Features/Hafenrichter. The picture of different herbal formulations is reproduced with permission of Alain Dex, Publiphoto Diffusion/Science Photo Library. The pictures of St John's wort and valerian are reproduced with permission of Glenis Moore/A-Z Botanical and A-Z Botanical. The picture of echinacea is reproduced with permission of NHPA/Stephen Krasemann. The picture of a Western herbalist is reproduced with permission of BMJ/Ulrike Preuss.

6 Homoeopathy

Background

Homoeopaths treat disease using very low dose preparations administered according to the principle that "like should be cured with like." Practitioners select a drug that would, if given to a healthy volunteer, cause the presenting symptoms of the patient. For example, the homoeopathic remedy *Allium cepa* is derived from the common onion. Contact with raw onions typically causes lacrimation, stinging and irritation around the eyes and nose, and clear nasal discharge. *Allium cepa* might be prescribed to patients with hay fever, especially if both nose and eyes are affected.

Other common homoeopathic medicines include those made from plants such as belladonna, arnica, and chamomile; minerals such as mercury and sulphur; animal products such as sepia (squid ink) and lachesis (snake venom); and, more rarely, biochemical substances such as histamine or human growth factor. The remedies are prepared by a process of serial dilution and succussion (vigorous shaking). The more times this process of dilution and succussion is performed, the greater the "potency" of the remedy.

Prescribing strategies in homoeopathy vary considerably. In what is often termed "classical" homoeopathy, practitioners attempt to identify the single medicine that corresponds to a patient's general "constitution"—a complex picture incorporating current illness, medical history, personality, and behaviour. Two patients with identical conventional diagnoses may receive very different homoeopathic medicines.

Other practitioners prescribe combinations of medicines ("complex homoeopathy") or prescribe on the basis of conventional diagnosis alone. There is currently insufficient evidence concerning the relative benefits of the different approaches to treatment.

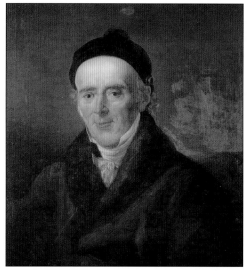

Samuel Hahnemann (1755-1843), the German physician who first described homoeopathy, began his pioneering experiments in the 1790s

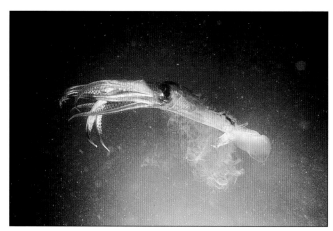

Homoeopathic medicines are made from various materials, including animal products such as sepia from squid ink

How can homoeopathy work?

It is well known that many homoeopathic medicines are ultramolecular—that is, they are diluted to such a degree that not even a single molecule of the original solute is likely to be present. As drug actions are conventionally understood in biochemical terms, homoeopathy presents an enormous intellectual challenge, if not a complete impasse. Many scientists have suggested that the clinical effects of homoeopathic medicines are solely due to the placebo effect. However, there have been rigorous, replicated, double blind, randomised trials showing significant differences between homoeopathic and placebo tablets.

The response to this has been mixed. Some people remain unconvinced by the evidence, claiming that there must be another explanation, such as methodological bias, for the results. Others point out that the evidence is very strong and argue that homoeopathic medicines must work by some, as yet undefined, biophysical mechanism. One possible explanation, currently being investigated, is that during serial dilution the complex interactions between the solvent (water) molecules are altered to retain a "memory" of the original solute material.

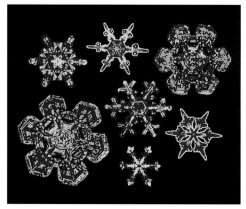

The complex lattice formations created by water molecules are thought by some to hold the key to understanding the mechanism by which homoeopathy might work

What happens during a treatment?

Homoeopaths' consultations for chronic conditions include an extremely detailed case history. Patients are asked to describe their medical history and current symptoms. Particular attention is paid to the "modalities" of presenting symptoms—that is, whether they change according to the weather, time of day, season, and so on. Information is also gathered about mood and behaviour, likes and dislikes, responses to stress, personality, and reactions to food. The overall aim of the history taking is to build up a "symptom picture" of the patient. This is matched with a "drug picture" described in the homoeopathic *Materia medica*. On this basis, one or more homoeopathic medicines are prescribed, usually in pill form. Sometimes treatment consists of only one or two doses. In other cases a regular daily dose is used.

Two to six weeks after the start of treatment, progress is reviewed and alterations made to remedy or dilution. A patient's initial symptom picture commonly matches more than one homoeopathic remedy, and follow up allows the practitioner to make an empirical judgment on whether a particular remedy was the correct one to prescribe. If the patient is doing well the practitioner may stop treatment and monitor progress. If symptoms recur the treatment may be repeated at the same or a higher potency. If the symptom picture has changed at follow up a different homoeopathic prescription may be given even though the conventional diagnosis remains unchanged.

Homoeopathic consultations in private practice may last over an hour, although many NHS general practitioners practise basic homoeopathy in 10-15 minute appointments. Many homoeopaths also recommend changes to diet and lifestyle, and some advise against vaccination (see section on safety below).

Therapeutic scope

Most of a typical homoeopath's caseload consists of chronic or recurrent conditions such as eczema, rheumatoid arthritis, fatigue disorders, asthma, migraine, dysmenorrhoea, irritable bowel syndrome, recurrent upper respiratory or urinary tract infections, and mood disorders. Homoeopaths also treat a substantial number of patients with ill defined illness that has not been given a conventional diagnosis. Children are much more commonly treated by homoeopaths than by other types of complementary practitioner.

Some homoeopaths say that few conditions are truly outside their remit, and the homoeopathic case literature includes treatment of complaints as diverse as tuberous sclerosis, infertility, myasthenia gravis, fear of flying, and cystic fibrosis. That said, opinions about what can be effectively treated by homoeopathy differ widely, even among homoeopaths, with medically trained practitioners generally being more conservative than non-medical ones. It is also used, often by self prescription, to treat various acute conditions such as the common cold, bruising, hay fever, and joint sprains.

Research evidence
Given the difficulties in understanding how homoeopathy may work, researchers have concentrated on establishing whether it is a placebo treatment. Current evidence suggests that this is probably not the case. A recent meta-analysis, published in the *Lancet*, examined over 100 randomised, placebo controlled trials and found an odds ratio of 2.45 (95% confidence interval 2.05 to 2.93) in favour of homoeopathy. The authors concluded that, even allowing for publication bias, "the results of our

Examples of "drug pictures" of commonly prescribed homoeopathic medicines

Aconite (*Aconitum napellus*)
Shock
- Sudden or violent onset
- Ailments from shock, fright, or fear
- Intense fear. Terror stricken. Predicts the time of death
- Restlessness with fear of death
- Ailments from exposure to cold, dry wind
- Worse with violent emotions, cold, night (especially around midnight)
- Better with open air, wine

Chamomile (*Matricaria chamomilla*)
Teething infant
- Child wants to be carried and is then more quiet
- Twitchings and convulsions during teething
- Frantic irritability with intolerance of pain
- Ugly, cross, uncivil, and quarrelsome
- Colic after anger
- Worse with anger, night, dentition, coffee
- Better with being carried, warm wet weather

Rhus toxicodendron
Joint pains worse with first movement and rest and better with motion
- Pain and stiffness worse in damp weather
- Irritability and restlessness at night, driving out of bed
- Back pains and stiffness compelling constant movement in bed
- Urticaria, vesicles. Cold air makes skin painful
- Asthma alternating with skin eruptions
- Worse with exposure to wet, cold, before storms, rest, first movement
- Better with heat, continued motion, rubbing, hot bath

Adapted from Leckridge 1997

Examples of symptomatic homoeopathic prescribing

Remedy	Condition
Cuprum	Leg cramps
Chamomile	Teething
Arnica	Bruising and trauma
Cantharis	Cystitis
Aconite	Croup
Colocynth	Infantile colic
Rhus tox.	Joint pain

Key studies of efficacy
Systematic reviews
- Kleijnen J, Knipschild P, ter Riet G. Clinical trials of homoeopathy. *BMJ* 1991;302:316-23
- Linde K, Clausius N, Ramirez G, Melchart D, Eitel F, Hedges LV, et al. Are the clinical effects of homeopathy placebo effects? A meta-analysis of placebo-controlled trials. *Lancet* 1997;350:834-43

Randomised controlled trials
- Reilly D, Taylor MA, Beattie NG, Campbell JH, McSharry C, Aitchison TC, et al. Is evidence for homoeopathy reproducible? *Lancet* 1994;344:1601-6

Laboratory studies
- Belon P, Cumps J, Ennis M, Mannaioni PF, Sainte-Laudy J, Roberfroid M, et al. Inhibition of human basophil degranulation by successive histamine dilutions: results of a European multi-centre trial. *Inflamm Res* 1999:48(suppl 1):S17-8
- Linde K, Jonas WB, Melchart D, Worku F, Wagner H, Eitel F. Critical review and meta-analysis of serial agitated dilutions in experimental toxicology. *Hum Exp Toxicol* 1994;13:481-92

meta-analysis are not compatible with the hypothesis that the clinical effects of homoeopathy are completely due to placebo."

The notorious Benveniste affair, which involved accusations of fraud and scientific misconduct after the publication of an in vitro experiment in *Nature*, continues to dampen enthusiasm for basic research in homoeopathy. None the less, some currently unreplicated laboratory studies have reported biological effects of homoeopathic medicines on animals, plants, and cells—some at ultramolecular dilutions.

Evidence is less clear on the effectiveness of homoeopathy as it is generally practised for the conditions that homoeopaths usually treat. Many trials have investigated treatment of an acute condition with a single remedy. This makes research easier but does not reflect the real world of homoeopathic clinical practice. For example, in the best known UK trial 144 patients with hay fever were randomised to receive either homoeopathically prepared grass pollen or placebo. Though there was a significant result in favour of homoeopathy, implications for clinical practice are unclear as most homoeopaths do not treat hay fever with homoeopathic grass pollen alone.

There is currently insufficient evidence that homoeopathy is clearly efficacious for any single clinical condition. For many of the conditions treated in homoeopathic practice—such as depression, fatigue, and eczema—randomised trials have not been undertaken. In addition, few of the existing studies of homoeopathy have been independently replicated.

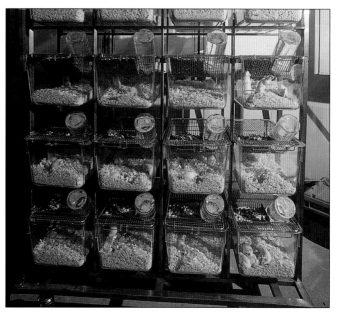

Laboratory experiments showing effects of homoeopathic medicines on animals provide evidence that the effects of homoeopathy are not entirely due to placebo

Safety of homoeopathy

Serious unexpected adverse effects of homoeopathic medicines are rare. "Aggravation reactions," when symptoms become acutely and transiently worse after starting homoeopathic treatment, have been described and are said by homoeopaths to be a good prognostic factor. They may cause concern, especially if patients and doctors are not adequately forewarned.

A potentially more serious issue is the belief of some practitioners that conventional drugs reduce the efficacy of homoeopathy. Serious adverse events have resulted from patients failing to comply with essential conventional treatments while using homoeopathy. Some, mainly non-medical, homoeopaths are also strongly against vaccination, although the official policy of the Society of Homoeopaths is to give patients information and choice and not to pressurise against immunisation. Homoeopaths may offer alternatives to vaccination. These have not been subjected to clinical trials and cannot therefore be recommended as an effective substitute.

There have been examples of homoeopathic medicines being adulterated with drugs, although this is extremely unlikely in the case of registered practitioners in Britain.

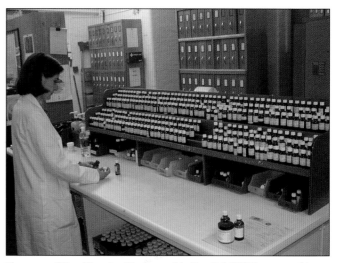

Some homoeopaths, mainly those without medical qualifications, believe that vaccination does more harm than good

Practitioners

About 1000 UK doctors practise homoeopathy, although fewer than half of these are full members of the Faculty of Homoeopathy. Many are general practitioners who have received only a basic training and who normally prescribe a limited number of remedies for specific acute conditions. Over 1500 homoeopaths without a conventional healthcare background are thought to practise in the United Kingdom.

Homoeopathy has been part of the NHS since its inception. There are currently five homoeopathic hospitals, of which the two largest, in Glasgow and London, have inpatient units. The hospitals provide a range of conventional and complementary treatments in addition to homoeopathy. Normal NHS

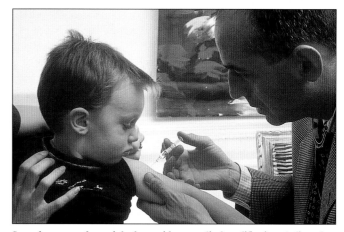

Pharmacy of Royal London Homoeopathic Hospital. NHS homoeopathic hospitals employ conventionally trained pharmacists, who have additional training in homoeopathy and sometimes herbal medicine. They dispense a range of complementary medicines which are prescribed by medically qualified practitioners

conditions apply: patients receive services free at the point of care, and the hospitals are reimbursed through block contracts with health authorities or extracontractual referrals. Some independent homoeopaths have had contracts with fundholding general practices and health authorities and have provided treatment for NHS patients.

Homoeopathic medicines can be purchased over the counter at chemists and health stores. They can also be prescribed on an FP10 form (GP10 in Scotland) by any doctor registered with the General Medical Council. About 10-20% of the UK population have bought homoeopathic products over the counter.

Homoeopathy is particularly popular in Europe: over 10 000 German and French doctors practise homoeopathy, and homoeopathic medicines constitute a substantial share of these countries' over the counter markets.

Training

The Faculty of Homoeopathy offers doctors a 40 hour course, approved for postgraduate education allowance, and an examination that lead to a primary care healthcare certificate. Intermediate and advanced courses are also available. The minimum entry requirement for the faculty's membership examination (MFHom) is 150-180 hours of study.

Training for homoeopaths without a medical background varies from three years part time to three years full time. Some training courses lead to university degrees in homoeopathy.

Regulation

The Faculty of Homoeopathy maintains a register of medical homoeopaths. The Society of Homoeopaths is the main regulatory body for practitioners without conventional healthcare qualifications and registers or licenses about 75% of homoeopathic practitioners in the United Kingdom.

Further reading

- Leckridge B. *Homoepathy in primary care*. Edinburgh: Churchill Livingstone, 1997
- Swayne J. *The homoeopathic method: implications for clinical practice and medical science*. Edinburgh: Churchill Livingstone, 1998

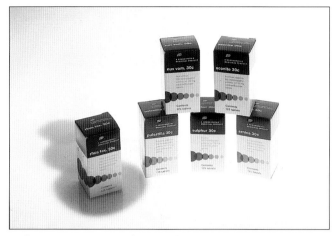

A wide range of homoeopathic preparations, usually of low potency, are available over the counter. Most are used for self medication on a simple, symptom matching basis

Addresses of regulatory bodies

Faculty of Homoeopathy
For medically trained homoeopaths
15 Clerkenwell Close, London EC1R 0AA. Tel: 020 7566 7800.
    Fax: 020 7566 7815. Email: info@trusthomeopathy.org

Society of Homoeopaths
Mainly for non-medically qualified homoeopaths
2 Artizan Road, Northampton NN1 4HU. Tel: 01604 621400.
    Fax: 01604 622622. Email: societyofhomoeopaths@btinternet.com
    URL: www.homoeopathy.org.uk

Key studies of efficacy

Systematic reviews
- Vickers AJ, Smith C. Homeopathic Oscillococcimum for preventing and treating influenza and influenza-like syndromes (protocol for a Cochrane Review). In: *The Cochrane Library*, **Issue 1**. Oxford: Update Software, 2000

Laboratory studies
- Hirst SJ, Hayes NA, Burridge J, Pearce FL, Foreman JC. Human basophil degranulation is not triggered by very dilute antiserum against human IgE. *Nature* 1993;**366**(6455): 525-7
- Anagnostatos GS, Pissis P, Viras K, Soutzidou M. Theory and experiments on high dilutions. In: Ernst E and Hahn EG (eds). *Homeopathy: a critical appraisal*, 1998 Oxford: Butterworth Heinemann

7 Hypnosis and relaxation therapies

A wide variety of complementary therapies claim to improve health by producing relaxation. Some use the relaxed state as a means of promoting psychological change. Others incorporate movement, stretches, and breathing exercises. Hypnosis, relaxation and "stress management" are found to a certain extent within conventional medicine. They are included here because they are generally not well taught in conventional medical curriculums and because of the overlap with other, more clearly complementary, therapies.

Techniques

Hypnosis

Hypnosis is the induction of a deeply relaxed state, with increased suggestibility and suspension of critical faculties. Once in this state, sometimes called a hypnotic trance, patients are given therapeutic suggestions to encourage changes in behaviour or relief of symptoms. For example, in a treatment to stop smoking a hypnosis practitioner might suggest that the patient will no longer find smoking pleasurable or necessary. Hypnosis for a patient with arthritis might include a suggestion that the pain can be turned down like the volume of a radio.

Some practitioners use hypnosis as an aid to psychotherapy. The rationale is that in the hypnotised state the conscious mind presents fewer barriers to effective psychotherapeutic exploration, leading to an increased likelihood of psychological insight.

Relaxation and meditation techniques

One well known example of a relaxation technique is known variously as sequential muscle relaxation (SMR), progressive relaxation, and Jacobson relaxation. The subject sits comfortably in a dark, quiet room. He or she then tenses a group of muscles, such as those in the right arm, holds the contraction for 15 seconds, and then releases it while breathing out. After a short rest, this sequence is repeated with another set of muscles. Gradually, different sets of muscle are combined.

The Mitchell method involves adopting body positions that are opposite to those associated with anxiety (fingers spread rather than hands clenched, for example). In autogenic training subjects concentrate on experiencing physical sensations, such as warmth and heaviness, in different parts of their bodies in a learnt sequence. Other methods encourage deepening and slowing the breath and a conscious attempt to let go of tension during exhalation.

Visualisation and imagery techniques are somewhat akin to hypnosis: the induction of a relaxed state followed by the use of suggestion. The main differences are that the suggestions are visual and usually generated by patients themselves. In cancer treatment, for example, patients may be asked to think of an image which represents their immune system killing off cancerous cells. One patient might imagine immune cells as sharks and the cancer cells as small fishes being eaten; another might think of a computer game in which the cancer cells are "zapped" by spaceships.

Meditation practice focuses on stilling or emptying the mind. Typically, meditators concentrate on their breath or a sound ("mantra") which they repeat to themselves. They may, alternatively, attempt to reach a state of "detached observation," in which they are aware of their environment but do not

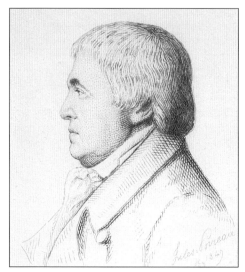

Franz Mesmer, 1734-1815, was responsible for the rise in popularity, and notoriety, of hypnosis ("mesmerism") in the 18th century

---

Definitions of terms relating to hypnosis

Hypnotic trance—A deeply relaxed state with increased suggestibility and suspension of critical faculties

Direct hypnotic suggestion—Suggestion made to a person in a hypnotic trance that alters behaviour or perception while the trance persists (for example, the suggestion that pain is not a problem for a woman under hypnosis during labour)

Post-hypnotic suggestion—Suggestion made to a person in a hypnotic trance that alters behaviour or perception after the trance ends (for example, the suggestion that in the future a patient will be able to relax at will and will no longer be troubled by panic attacks)

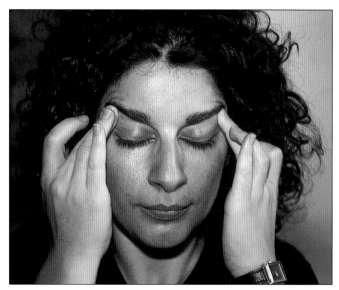

Many relaxation techniques aim to increase awareness of areas of chronic unconscious muscle tension. They often involve a conscious attempt to release and relax during exhalation

become involved in thinking about it. In meditation the body remains alert and in an upright poition.

Yoga practice involves postures, breathing exercises, and meditation aimed at improving mental and physical functioning. Some practitioners understand yoga in terms of traditional Indian medicine, with the postures improving the flow of "prana" energy around the body. Others see yoga in more conventional terms of muscle stretching and mental relaxation.

Tai chi is a gentle system of exercises originating from China. The best known example is the "solo form," a series of slow and graceful movements that follow a set pattern. It is said to improve strength, balance, and mental calmness. Qigong (pronounced "chi kung") is another traditional Chinese system of therapeutic exercises. Practitioners teach meditation, physical movements, and breathing exercises to improve the flow of Qi, the Chinese term for body energy.

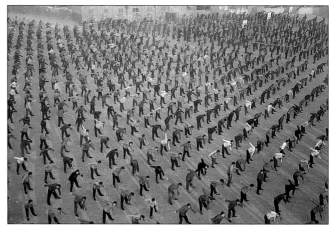
In China many people practise tai chi for health promotion on a daily basis

What happens during a treatment?

Hypnosis
In hypnosis, patients normally see practitioners by themselves for a course of hourly or half hourly treatments. Some general practitioners and other medical specialists use hypnosis as part of their regular clinical work and follow a longer initial consultation with standard 10-15 minute appointments. Patients can be given a post-hypnotic suggestion that enables them to induce self hypnosis after the treatment course is completed. Some practitioners undertake group hypnosis, treating up to a dozen patients at a time—for example, teaching self hypnosis to antenatal groups as preparation for labour.

Relaxation and meditation techniques
Most relaxation techniques need to be practised daily. Typically, patients learn a relaxation technique over the course of eight weekly classes, each lasting an hour or so. Between classes, they practise by themselves for 15 to 30 minutes a day. After the course is over, patients are encouraged to continue on their own, though they may take further classes to learn advanced techniques or to maintain group support. Methods such as sequential muscle relaxation are learnt relatively readily: yoga, tai chi, and meditation can take years to master completely.

Most relaxation techniques are enjoyable, and many healthy individuals practise them without having particular health problems. Relaxation classes can also play a social function.

Unlike in many other complementary therapies, practitioners of relaxation techniques do not make diagnoses. They may use the conventional diagnoses as described by the patient to tailor the prescribed programme appropriately. However, in many cases the method of treatment does not depend on a precise diagnosis.

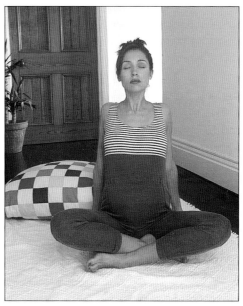
Self hypnosis can be taught to pregnant women as preparation for labour

Therapeutic scope

The primary uses of hypnosis and relaxation techniques are in anxiety, in disorders with a strong psychological component (such as asthma and irritable bowel syndrome), and in conditions that can be modulated by levels of arousal (such as pain). They are also commonly used in programmes for stress management.

Research evidence
There is good evidence from randomised controlled trials that both hypnosis and relaxation techniques can reduce anxiety, particularly that related to stressful situations such as receiving

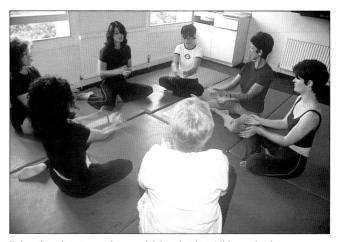
Relaxation classes can play a social function in addition to having therapeutic benefits

chemotherapy. They are also effective for panic disorders and insomnia, particularly when integrated into a package of cognitive therapy (including, for example, sleep hygiene). A systematic review has found that hypnosis enhances the effects of cognitive behavioural therapy for conditions such as phobia, obesity, and anxiety.

Randomised controlled trials support the use of various relaxation techniques for treating both acute and chronic pain, although two recent systematic reviews suggest that methodological flaws may compromise the reliability of these findings. Randomised trials have shown hypnosis to be of value in asthma and in irritable bowel syndrome, yoga to be of benefit in asthma, and tai chi to help in reducing falls and fear of falls in elderly people. There is evidence from systematic reviews that hypnosis and relaxation techniques are probably not of general benefit in stopping smoking or substance misuse or in treating hypertension.

Relaxation and hypnosis are often used in cancer patients. There is strong evidence from randomised trials of the effectiveness of hypnosis and relaxation for cancer related anxiety, pain, nausea, and vomiting, particularly in children. Some practitioners also claim that hypnosis or relaxation techniques, particularly those incorporating visualisation, can prolong life. Though some positive randomised trials of psychosocial interventions (which generally include psychotherapy or cognitive-behavioural therapy as well as hypnosis and/or relaxation) have been published, there is currently insufficient evidence to support this claim.

Safety

Adverse events resulting from relaxation techniques seem to be extremely uncommon. Though rare, there have been reports of basilar or vertebral artery occlusion after yoga postures that put particular strain on the neck. Sequential muscle relaxation should be avoided by people with poorly controlled cardiovascular disease as abdominal tensing can cause the Valsalva response. In patients with a history of psychosis or epilepsy there have been reports of further acute episodes after deep and prolonged meditation.

Hypnosis or deep relaxation, including Qi Gong, can sometimes exacerbate psychological problems—for example, by retraumatising those with post-traumatic disorders or by inducing "false memories" in psychologically vulnerable individuals. Concerns have also been raised that it can bring on a latent psychosis, although the evidence is inconclusive. Hypnosis should be undertaken only by appropriately trained, experienced, and regulated practitioners. It should be avoided in established or borderline psychosis and personality disorders, and hypnotherapists should be competent at recognising and referring patients in these states.

Practice

Relaxation techniques are often integrated into other healthcare practices. For example, they may be included in programmes of cognitive behavioural therapy in pain clinics or occupational therapy in psychiatric units. Many different complementary therapists, such as osteopaths and massage therapists, may include some relaxation techniques in their work. Some nurses use relaxation techniques in the acute setting, such as in preparation for surgery. A small number of general practices offer regular classes in relaxation, yoga, or tai chi.

Key studies of efficacy

Systematic reviews
- Carroll D, Seers K. Relaxation for the relief of chronic pain: a systematic review. *J Adv Nurs* 1998;27:476-87
- Eisenberg DM, Delbanco TL, Berkey CS, Kaptchuk TJ, Kupelnick B, Kuhl J, et al. Cognitive behavioral techniques for hypertension: are they effective? *Ann Intern Med* 1993;118:964-72
- Kirsch I, Montgomery G, Sapirstein G. Hypnosis as an adjunct to cognitive-behavioral psychotherapy: a meta-analysis. *J Consult Clin Psychol* 1995;63:214-20

Randomised controlled trials
- Harvey RF, Hinton RA, Gunary RM, Barry RE. Individual and group hypnotherapy in treatment of refractory irritable bowel syndrome. *Lancet* 1989;i:424-5
- Nagarathna R, Nagendra HR. Yoga for bronchial asthma: a controlled study. *BMJ* 1985;291:1077-9
- Spiegel D, Bloom JR, Kraemer HC, Gottheil E. Effect of psychosocial treatment on survival of patients with metastatic cancer. *Lancet* 1989;2:888-91

Other
- NIH Technology Assessment Panel on Integration of Behavioral and Relaxation Approaches into the Treatment of Chronic Pain and Insomnia. Integration of behavioral and relaxation approaches into the treatment of chronic pain and insomnia. *JAMA* 1996;276:313-8

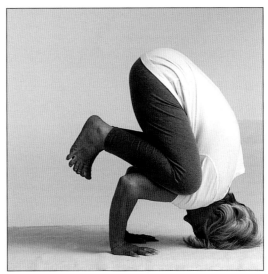

Though rare, cases of basilar or vertebral artery occlusion have been reported after certain yoga positions that put stress on the neck

Registering and training organisations

British Society of Medical and Dental Hypnosis
For doctors and dentists only
17 Keppel View Road, Kinberworth, Rotherham, S Yorks S61 2AR.
Tel/Fax: 0700 560309. Email: nat.office@bsmdh.org.
URL: www.bsmdh.org

British Society of Medical and Dental Hypnosis—Scotland
PO Box 1007, Glasgow, G31 2LE. Tel: 0141 556 1606.
Fax: 0141 551 9104

British Society for Experimental and Clinical Hypnosis
For doctors, dentists and psychologists only
Department of Clinical Oncology, Derbyshire Royal Infirmary, London Road, Derby DE1 2QY. Tel: 01332 766791.
Fax: 01332 776863. Email: phyllis@alden-residence.demon.co.uk

Yoga Biomedical Trust
4th Floor, Royal London Homoeopathic Hospital, London WC1N 3HR. Tel: 020 7419 7195. Fax: 020 7419 7196.
Email: yogabio.med@virgin.net

Regulation

The practice of many relaxation techniques is poorly regulated, and standards of practice and training are variable. This situation is unsatisfactory, but, given the relatively benign nature of many relaxation techniques, this variation in standards presents usually more of a problem of ensuring effective treatment and good professional conduct rather than one of avoiding adverse effects.

For hypnosis and deeper relaxation techniques, poor regulation is a more serious issue. The large number of hypnotherapy registers and the lack of a single regulating body makes selecting a practitioner difficult. Hypnotherapists with a conventional healthcare background (such as psychologists, doctors, dentists, and nurses) will be regulated by their conventional professional regulatory bodies. Some of the organisations registering hypnotherapists without a conventional background are member associations of the British Complementary Medicine Association (see third article of this series).

When hypnosis is used as a psychotherapeutic or psychoanalytic tool practitioners require appropriate training and experience in clinical psychology, counselling, or psychotherapy. Hypnotherapists who practise in this way should be members of the British Psychological Society, the British Association of Counselling, or the United Kingdom Council of Psychotherapy.

Training

The British Society for Medical and Dental Hypnosis and the British Society of Experimental and Clinical Hypnosis run basic, intermediate, and advanced courses for doctors and other conventionally trained healthcare professionals. Both organisations and the Section of Hypnosis and Phsychosomatic Medicine of the Royal Society of Medicine hold regular scientific meetings. There is no standard training in hypnosis for practitioners without a conventional healthcare background.

Training in teaching relaxation techniques is provided through various routes from self teaching, through apprenticeships, to a number of short courses. Many yoga centres run courses to train yoga teachers. The Yoga Biomedical Trust also trains yoga therapists, who see patients individually and work on specific health problems.

Other useful addresses

Royal Society of Medicine Section on Hypnosis and Psychosomatic Medicine
For doctors, dentists and veterinary surgeons
1 Wimpole Street, London W1N 8AE. Tel: 020 7290 2986.
  Fax: 020 7290 2989. Email: hypnosis@roysocmed.ac.uk

British Psychological Society (BPS)
St Andrews House, 48 Princess Road East, Leicester LE1 7DR
  Tel: 0116 254 9568. Fax: 0116 247 0787. URL: www.bps.org.uk

British Association of Counselling (BAC)
1 Regent Place, Rugby, Warwickshire CV21 2PJ. Tel: 01788 550899.
  Fax: 01788 562189. URL: www.counselling.co.uk

United Kingdom Council of Psychotherapy (UKCP)
167-9 Great Portland Street, London W1N 5FB. Tel: 020 7436 3002.
  Fax: 020 7436 3013. URL: www.ukcp.org.uk

British Complementary Medicine Association (BCMA)
249 Fosse Road South, Leicester LE3 1AE. Tel: 0116 282 5511

Further reading

- Waxman D. *Medical-dental hypnosis*. London: Balliere Tindall, 1988
- Karle H, Boys J. *Hypnotherapy: a practical handbook*. London: Free Association Books, reprinted 1996
- Siegel B. *Love, medicine and miracles*. London: Arrow, 1989

8   The manipulative therapies: osteopathy and chiropractic

Osteopathy and chiropractic share a common origin. Their roots can be found in folk traditions of "bone setting," and both were systematised in the late 19th century in the United States: Daniel D Palmer, the founder of chiropractic, is said to have met with Andrew Taylor Still, the founder of osteopathy, before setting up his own school. The therapies remain relatively similar, and many textbooks and journals are relevant to both. The term "manipulative therapy" refers to both osteopathy and chiropractic. This chapter will describe manipulative therapy as practised in the UK. Readers should be aware that osteopathy and chiropractic are somewhat different in the USA, in particular, osteopaths have similar licensing to mainstream doctors and use conventional interventions, such as medication, in their work.

Background

Osteopathy and chiropractic are therapies of the musculoskeletal system: practitioners work with bones, muscles, and connective tissue, using their hands to diagnose and treat abnormalities of structure and function.

The best known technique is the "high velocity thrust," a short, sharp motion usually applied to the spine. This manoeuvre is designed to release structures with a restricted range of movement. High velocity thrusts often produce the sound of joint "cracking," which is associated with manipulative therapy. There are various methods of delivering a high velocity thrust. Chiropractors are more likely to push on vertebrae with their hands, whereas osteopaths tend use the limbs to make levered thrusts. That said, osteopathic and chiropractic techniques are converging, and much of their therapeutic repertoire is shared.

Practitioners also use a range of soft tissue techniques that do not involve high velocity thrusts. For example, the "muscle energy techniques" (known as "proprioceptive neuromuscular facilitation" by physiotherapists) make use of post-isometric relaxation to increase restricted ranges of movement.

Osteopaths and chiropractors may also use what are termed "functional techniques," such as treating hip pain by applying a gentle, prolonged pull to the leg while slowly rotating it in the hip joint. If a restriction is detected, however slight, the leg is held at the point of restriction until a release of muscle tension occurs. Techniques like these are based on an understanding of subtle neuromuscular behaviour, which conforms to mainstream theory. In practice, they also rely on finely developed palpatory skills.

Some osteopaths also practise a technique known as cranial osteopathy or craniosacral therapy. Practitioners place their hands on the cranium and sacrum and gently handle the bones of the skull. They say that, by feeling for and working with subtle rhythmic pulsations of the cerebrospinal fluid, they can correct disturbances in the neuromuscular system. There are some therapists, usually known as craniosacral therapists, who use similar techniques but who do not have an osteopathic background.

A relatively recent branch of chiropractic, the McTimoney school, has developed some of its own manipulative techniques that do not place as great an emphasis on high velocity thrusts as do osteopathy and mainstream chiropractic.

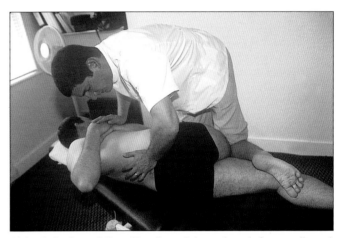

High velocity thrust delivered by a levered thrust, the technique usually used by osteopaths

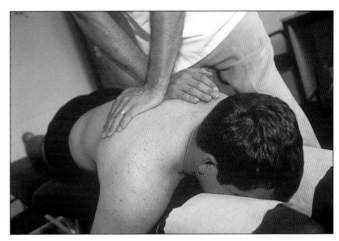

High velocity thrust given as a direct thrust on the spine, as favoured by chiropractors

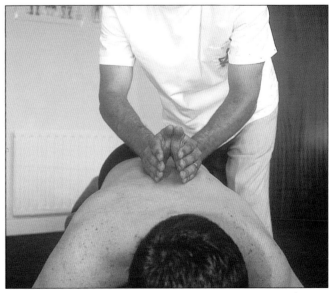

Chiropractors and osteopaths may use soft tissue techniques to increase a joint's range of movement or relieve muscular spasm

With the exception of cranial osteopathy, many of the treatment methods used by osteopaths and chiropractors are similar to techniques used by those physiotherapists with additional training in manipulative therapy. From a general practitioner's perspective, there are few important practical differences between the three types of practitioner.

What happens during a treatment?

Manipulative therapists take a history, palpate for significant changes in muscle tension and skin circulation, and look for any restricted movements in order to diagnose musculoskeletal abnormalities and "neuromuscular dysfunction" (such as "trigger points" or signs of "pain-spasm cycles"). Chiropractors may use x rays to assist diagnosis, whereas osteopaths do so largely only for the purposes of excluding serious pathology.

A typical treatment session lasts 15-30 minutes, although first consultations may take longer. A variety of the techniques described above will be used. Not more than four high velocity thrusts are usually given in a single treatment session. A course of chiropractic treatment for back pain might consist of six sessions, initially frequent and then at weekly intervals. Osteopaths are more likely than chiropractors to treat on an "as needed" basis.

Therapeutic scope

Both osteopathy and chiropractic were originally regarded as complete systems of medicine. For example, Andrew Taylor Still treated infectious diseases and blindness among a range of conditions. Interestingly, the treatment of back problems features only rarely in his writings. Similarly, early chiropractors believed that most diseases could be attributed to misalignments of the spine and were therefore amenable to treatment with chiropractic.

Contemporary practitioners have moved away from this position and concentrate primarily on musculoskeletal disorders. Low back pain is the most common presenting complaint. Guidelines from the Royal College of General Practitioners recommend physical therapy (any of the manipulative techniques) within six weeks of the start of persisting uncomplicated back pain.

Other conditions often seen include neck and shoulder pain, sports injuries, repetitive strain disorders, and headache. Practitioners also treat various conditions such as arthritis; although they cannot affect disease pathology or progression, they claim to be able to treat secondary symptoms such as pain from associated muscle spasm. Cranial osteopathy has a particular reputation for treating children with conditions such as infantile colic, constant crying, and behavioural problems.

Research evidence

There is considerable evidence from randomised controlled trials of the effectiveness of spinal manipulation for back and neck pain. Although this evidence is largely positive, it has been criticised for failing to exclude non-specific effects of treatment.

In the best known UK trial 741 patients with low back pain were randomised to chiropractic or hospital outpatient care. In both groups the treating practitioners were free to treat patients as they saw fit. The authors concluded that "chiropractic almost certainly confers worthwhile, long term benefit." However, a recent systematic review of this and similar trials highlights methodological weaknesses, such as the fact that commonly used outcome measures such as pain and disability scores are assessed by patients and therefore unblinded.

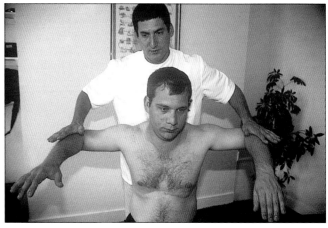

Palpatory assessment of areas of muscle spasm and tenderness, restricted joint movements, local differences in skin temperature, and sweat gland activity are all important in making a diagnosis and planning treatment

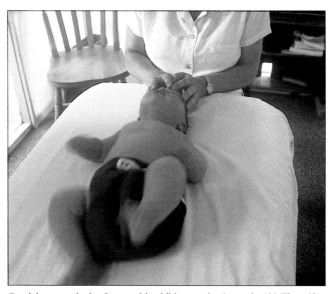

Cranial osteopathy is often used in children under 6 months old. The self limiting nature of many infantile problems (such as colic and irregular sleep patterns) means that evaluation by randomised controlled trials is essential

Key studies of efficacy

Systematic reviews
- Koes BW, Assendelft WJ, van der Heijen GJMG, Bouter LM, Knipschild PG. Spinal manipulation and mobilisation for back and neck pain: a blinded review. *BMJ* 1991;303:1298-303
- Koes BW, Assendelft WJ, van der Heijen GJMG, Bouter LM. Spinal manipulation for low back pain. An updated systematic review of randomised clinical trials. *Spine* 1996;21:2860-71

Randomised controlled trials
- Balon J, Aker PD, Crowther ER, Danielson C, Cox PG, O'Shaughnessy D, et al. A comparison of active and simulated chiropractic manipulation as adjunctive treatment for childhood asthma. *N Engl J Med* 1998;339:1013-20
- Meade TW, Dyer S, Browne W, Frank AO. Randomised comparison of chiropractic and hospital outpatient management for low back pain: results from extended follow up. *BMJ* 1995;311:349-51
- Meade TW, Dyer S, Browne W, Townsend J, Frank AO. Low back pain of mechanical origin: randomised comparison of chiropractic and hospital outpatient treatment. *BMJ* 1990;300:1431-7
- Koes BW, Bouter LM, van Mameren H, Essers AH, Verstegen GM, Hofhuizen DM, et al. Randomised clinical trial of manipulative therapy and physiotherapy for persistent back and neck complaints: results of one year follow up. *BMJ* 1992;304:601-5

In one trial that did involve blinded assessment of outcome, patients with back or neck pain were randomised to routine general practitioner care, placebo (deactivated heat treatment), physiotherapy, or manipulation. Physiotherapy and manipulation were superior to placebo and general practitioner care after six weeks, and manipulation was superior to physiotherapy at one year follow up.

In addition to effects on back and neck pain, randomised trials have also indicated that manipulative treatment is beneficial for headache, including migraine. However, the number of studies is small, so further work to confirm these results is needed. There is little or no reliable evidence of beneficial effects for many of the other musculoskeletal conditions that are commonly treated.

Apart from dysmenorrhoea, for which a small number of trials have shown a positive effect, current evidence suggests that manipulative therapy is not of benefit for problems related to smooth muscles or viscera, such as asthma and hypertension.

There has been little research on cranial osteopathy or McTimoney chiropractic.

Safety of osteopathy and chiropractic

The most important potential adverse effects of osteopathy and chiropractic are stroke and spinal cord injury after cervical manipulation. Estimates of such severe adverse events vary widely, ranging from 1 in 20 000 patients undergoing cervical manipulation to 1 per million procedures. In recent years the osteopathic and chiropractic professions have shown greater appreciation of the risks of cervical manipulation, and it is possible that improved practice is leading to a reduction in the rate of severe complications.

More common adverse effects (25-50% of all patients) are mild pain or discomfort at the site of manipulation, slight headache, and fatigue; 75% or more of such complaints resolve within 24 hours. Contraindications to various manipulative techniques have been developed by the appropriate professional bodies, and practitioners are trained to screen patients and assess individual risk factors. Even when some techniques, such as high velocity thrusts, are contraindicated, other manipulative treatments may be safe.

Practitioners

Osteopathy and chiropractic are almost exclusively based in the community and in the private sector. Many practitioners work alone, often from converted rooms in their own homes. Others work in group clinics, in multidisciplinary practices, or in general practices. Some independent manipulative practitioners have established contracts with health authorities, fundholding practices, or primary care groups. Most private health insurance schemes now offer some cover for manipulative treatment.

Regulation
Osteopathy and chiropractic are the only two complementary therapies that are regulated by statute. Two acts of parliament passed in the mid-1990s established a General Osteopathic Council and a General Chiropractic Council with the aim of regulating the professions by the millennium. These organisations operate in a similar way to the General Medical Council and have the authority to remove practitioners from the register in disciplinary hearings.

Training
Most osteopaths take a four year, full time course leading to a BSc degree (BOst). Chiropractors undertake a four to five year, full

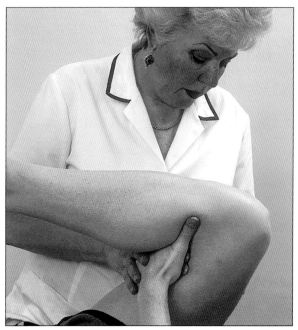

Many physiotherapists use manipulative techniques similar to those of chiropractors and osteopaths

Contraindications to high velocity thrusts

Absolute	Relative	No contraindication
Acute inflammatory arthropathies	Spondylolisthesis with ongoing slippage	Subacute inflammatory arthropathies
Acute fracture or dislocation	Articular hypermobility	Osteoarthritis
Ligament rupture and instability	Post-surgical joints with clinical signs of acute inflammation or instability	Spondylolisthesis with no change in slippage
Unstable odontoid peg	Demineralisation	Post-surgical joints with no signs of instability
Infection	Benign bone tumours	Acute injuries of soft and bony tissues
Vertebrobasilar arterial insufficiency	Anticoagulants	Scoliosis
Aneurysm		
Acute myelopathy		
Acute cauda equina syndrome		

Based on the Mercy guidelines from the proceedings of the Mercy Center Consensus Conference, Burlingham CA, USA, 1992

Regulatory bodies and sources of further information

General Osteopathic Council
Osteopathy House, 176 Tower Bridge Road, London SE1 3LU.
Tel: 020 7357 6655. Fax: 020 7357 0011.
Email: info@osteopathy.org.uk. URL: www.osteopathy.org.uk

General Chiropractic Council
Register opened 15 June 1999
3rd Floor North, 344-354 Gray's Inn Road, London WC1X 8BP.
Tel: 020 7713 5155 (for queries about regulation 0845 601 1796).
Fax: 020 7713 5844. Email: enquiries@gcc-uk.freeserve.co.uk

Manipulative Association of Chartered Physiotherapists
c/o Professional Affairs, Chartered Society of Physiotherapists,
14 Bedford Row, London WC1R 4ED. Tel: 020 7242 1941.
Fax: 020 7306 6611

time training, which includes a BSc in human sciences and chiropractic and a year of postgraduate training in an approved practice, leading to a diploma in chiropractic (DC). McTimoney and McTimoney Corley practitioners complete a four year, part time course. Biological and clinical sciences form a substantial component of all these training courses. Sometimes chiropractors are referred to as "doctors of chiropractic."

Several organisations run training courses in manipulative techniques specifically for conventional healthcare practitioners. The Manipulative Association of Chartered Physiotherapists runs and accredits postgraduate training in manipulation for physiotherapists. The British Institute of Musculoskeletal Medicine runs courses for medically qualified practitioners but is not a regulatory body. The London College of Osteopathic Medicine organises a one year, full time osteopathic training course for registered medical practitioners.

The pictures of manipulative techniques and of cranial osteopathy are reproduced with permission of BMJ/Ulrike Preuss. The picture of a physiotherapist is reproduced with permission of Science Photo Library.

Educational organisations for doctors

British Institute of Musculoskeletal Medicine
27 Green Lane, Northwood, Middlesex HA6 2PX. Tel/Fax: 01923 220999. Email: BIMM@compuserve.com

Society of Orthopaedic Medicine
c/o Amanda Sherwood, administrator. Tel: 01454 610255
   URL: www.soc-ortho-med.org

London College of Osteopathic Medicine
8-10 Boston Place, London NW1 6QH. Tel: 020 7262 5250. Fax: 020 7723 7492

Further reading
- Burn L. *A manual of medical manipulation.* Newbury: Petroc Press, 1998
- DiGiovanna EL, Schiowitz S, Dowling D. *An osteopathic approach to diagnosis and treatment.* Plymouth: Lippincott Raven, 1996
- Kaptchuk TJ, Eisenberg DM. Chiropractic: origins, controversies and contributions. *Arch Intern Med* 1998;158:2215-24

9 Massage therapies

Therapeutic massage is the manipulation of the soft tissue of whole body areas to bring about generalised improvements in health, such as relaxation or improved sleep, or specific physical benefits, such as relief of muscular aches and pains.

Background

Almost all cultures have developed systems of therapeutic massage. Massage techniques play an important part in traditional Chinese and Indian medical care. European massage was systematised in the early 18th century by Per Hendrik Ling, who developed what is now known as Swedish massage.

Ling believed that vigorous massage could bring about healing by improving the circulation of the blood and lymph. In the past 20-30 years complementary therapists have adapted Swedish massage so as to place greater emphasis on the psychological and spiritual aspects of treatment. Benefits of massage are now described more in terms such as "calmness" or "wholeness" than in terms of loosening stiff joints or improving blood flow. In contrast to the vigorous and standardised treatment recommended by Ling, current massage techniques are more gentle, calming, flowing, and intuitive.

Several techniques derive from traditions separate from European massage. In reflexology, areas of the foot are believed to correspond to the organs or structures of the body. Damage or disease in an organ is reflected in the corresponding region, or "reflex zone," of the foot. When this is palpated the patient is said to experience pain or pricking, no matter how gently pressure is applied. Reflexology treatment consists of massage of the disordered reflex zones.

In aromatherapy, oils derived from plants ("essential oils") are added to a base massage oil, which acts as a lubricant during treatment. Although often used purely for their smell, the oils are claimed to have a wide range of medicinal properties, including effects on wound healing, infection, blood circulation, and digestion. They are said to act both pharmacologically, by absorption into the blood through the skin, and by olfactory stimulation. Many massage practitioners use essential oils without claiming to be practising aromatherapy.

Various other complementary disciplines are primarily touch based or have a substantial touch component (see box).

What happens during a treatment?

Massage treatment takes a variety of forms and may last anywhere between 15 and 90 minutes. Treatment follows a case history, which is usually relatively short compared with other complementary therapies but which varies in length depending on the patient's condition and the indications for massage. While giving a standard massage, practitioners will also gather palpatory information, which helps tailor treatment to individual needs. For example, a practitioner will devote extra time to massage an area of increased muscle tension.

The patient is ideally treated unclothed, on a specially designed massage couch. This normally incorporates soft but firm padding and a hole for the face. The treatment room is kept warm and quiet. Soft music may sometimes be played.

Practitioners generally treat the whole body, using oil to help their hands move over the patient's body. A variety of

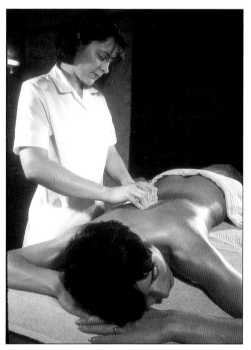

A typical massage treatment session

Examples of other predominantly touch based therapies

Rolfing *Structural integration* *Hellerwork*	Treatments which use deep pressure massage to improve function of muscular system
Alexander technique *Feldenkrais*	Educational systems incorporating exercises and hands-on therapy designed to improve posture, movement, and function
Bioenergetics	Massage to aid the psychotherapeutic process
"Bodywork"	Any combination of the above

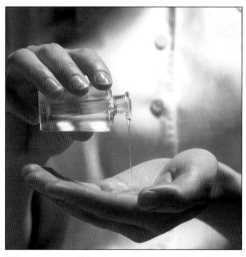

UK massage practitioners usually use an oil, such as sweet almond oil, as a lubricant. Elsewhere in Europe, soap or talcum powder are sometimes used instead

strokes are used, including effleurage, petrissage, kneading, and friction (see box). Massage practitioners who treat sports injuries and musculoskeletal disorders may incorporate techniques derived from physiotherapy, osteopathy, and chiropractic. These include deep massage, passive and active stretching, and muscle energy techniques (in which the patient moves against resistance from the practitioner).

Massage can be adapted to the constraints of conventional health settings by limiting work to the head, hands, feet, or back or even by giving a neck and shoulder rub through clothes with the patient sitting in a chair.

Patients usually find massage to be a deeply relaxing and pleasurable experience. Some techniques include strong pressure, which can cause painful sensations, but these are usually short lived.

Therapeutic scope

Massage is mainly used to promote relaxation, treat painful muscular conditions, and reduce anxiety (often described in terms of "relief from stress"). Practitioners also claim to bring about short term improvements in sleep disorders and pain, conditions known to be exacerbated by anxiety, and massage is widely used for these indications.

Massage is also claimed to have more global effects on health. Practitioners and patients report that massage improves self image in conditions such as physical disabilities and terminal illnesses. This may result in part from the feelings of general wellbeing that are commonly reported after massage. Touch itself is likely to be therapeutic, particularly in those with limited opportunities for physical contact, such as patients without intimate friends or family or with painful physical conditions.

Massage has also been said to help patients feel cared for. Patients may be more ready to discuss and deal with difficult psychological issues once they are less anxious, feel better about themselves, and have come to trust their care providers. Practitioners say that this is one of the reasons why massage can be an important stepping stone to effective counselling, for example, in managing mental health problems or addiction.

Massage has been used to foster communication and relationships in several other settings. In work with children with profound disabilities, where touch may be a primary means of communication, massage techniques have been incorporated into the everyday activities of care workers. Similarly, some midwives run "baby massage" groups where new mothers are taught massage as a means of improving their relationship with their children.

Practitioners of reflexology claim that, in addition to the relaxation and non-specific effects of massage, they can bring about more specific changes in health. One classic reflexology text, for example, includes case histories of ataxia, osteoarthritis, and epilepsy. Similarly, some aromatherapists report benefits in conditions as diverse as infertility, acne, diabetes, and hay fever.

Research evidence
To date, most of the clinical trials of massage have focused on psychological outcomes of treatment. Good evidence from randomised trials indicates that massage reduces anxiety scores in the short term in settings as varied as intensive care, psychiatric institutions, hospices, and occupational health. There is more limited evidence that these anxiety reductions are cumulative over time. Practitioners claim that giving patients a concrete experience of relaxation through massage can facilitate their use of self help relaxation techniques. This has yet

Techniques used in massage
Effleurage—Gentle stroking along the length of a muscle
Petrissage—Pressure applied across the width of a muscle
Friction—Deep massage applied by circular motions of the thumbs or fingertips
Kneading—Squeezing across the width of a muscle
Hacking—Light slaps or karate chops

Reports of psychological benefits of massage
Patient in primary care—"I was very surprised after the first massage that I had been able to bring into the open all these fears and feelings. I most certainly would have been far less forthcoming and far less frank in a situation of psychotherapy—i.e. sitting, fully dressed, face to face with a counsellor"
Patient with AIDS—"It was wonderful to be touched by someone who wasn't wearing gloves"
Patient with physical disability—"When I was being massaged it felt like a stroke up my back was traversing three countries. Massage made me aware of the splits and divisions in me. I certainly gain self acceptance through touch"
Patient with mental ill health—"Massage showed me that I can let go and nothing terrible will happen"

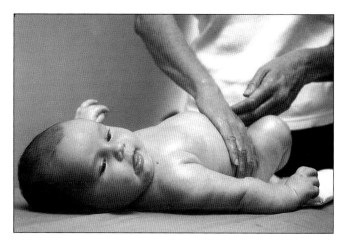
Baby massage is one way of encouraging physical interaction and stimulating the developing relationship between parent and child

Key studies of efficacy
Systematic review
- Vickers A, Ohlsson A, Lacy JB, Horsley A. Massage therapy for premature and/or low birth-weight infants to improve weight gain and/or to decrease hospital length of stay. In: Cochrane Collaboration. *The Cochrane Library.* Issue 3. Oxford: Update Software, 1998

Randomised controlled trials
- Field T, Morrow C, Valdeon C, Larson S, Kuhn C, Schanberg S. Massage reduces anxiety in child and adolescent psychiatric patients. *J Am Acad Child Adolesc Psychiatry* 1992;31:125-31
- Stevensen C. The psychophysiological effects of aromatherapy massage following cardiac surgery. *Complement Ther Med* 1994; 2:27-35
- Wilkinson S. Aromatherapy and massage in palliative care. *Int J Palliative Nurs* 1995;1:21-30

to be evaluated. The evidence that massage can lead to improved sleep and reduce pain remains anecdotal.

Some evidence supports the more "traditional" effects of massage such as improved circulation and decreased muscle tension. However, no reliable data link these changes to clinically worthwhile benefits such as relief of musculoskeletal pain, increased mobility, or improved athletic performance.

Randomised trials have provided some evidence that massage in premature infants is associated with objective outcomes such as more rapid weight gain and development. Many other anecdotal benefits of massage are more subtle and have not been subjected to randomised controlled trials.

There are very few clinical trials showing that any massage technique can have specific effects on conditions such as osteoarthritis, epilepsy, infertility, or diabetes. Very few trials have evaluated the relative advantages of different massage techniques.

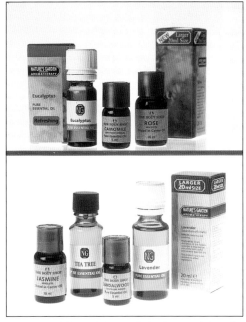

Massage on a hospital ward: foot massage has been shown to reduce anxiety even in highly stressful settings

Safety of massage techniques

Most massage techniques have a low risk of adverse effects. Cases reported in the literature are extremely rare and have usually involved techniques that are unusual in the United Kingdom, such as extremely vigorous massage.

Contraindications to massage are based largely on common sense (for example, avoiding friction on burns or massage in a limb with deep vein thrombosis) rather than empirical data. Massage after myocardial infarction is controversial, although studies have shown that gentle massage is only a moderate physiological stimulus that does not cause undue strain on the heart. There is no evidence that massage in patients with cancer increases metastatic spread, although direct firm pressure over sites of active tumour should generally be avoided.

Considerable concern has been raised about the safety of the oils used in aromatherapy. Although essential oils are pharmacologically active, and in some cases potentially carcinogenic in high concentrations, adverse events directly attributable to them are extremely rare. This may be because in practice the oils are used externally and in low doses (concentrations of 1-3%). However, the lack of a formal reporting scheme for adverse events in aromatherapy means that the safety of essential oils has not been conclusively established.

Massage obviously involves close physical contact. To minimise the risks of unprofessional behaviour in this situation, patients should ensure that practitioners are registered with an appropriate regulatory body.

More research is needed on both the therapeutic benefits and the safety implications of using essential oils in massage. However, the doses used are low, and problems seem to be extremely rare

Practice

Like many complementary therapies, massage is usually practised in private in the community. It is also found in conventional health settings, in particular in hospices and in units for learning disability and mental disorders. Massage in these settings is often practised by nurses or by unpaid practitioner volunteers, and much practice is informal, such as a head and neck rub for a distressed patient. However, an increasing number of professional massage practitioners are now employed in NHS hospitals and general practices.

Regulation
Practitioners of massage therapies are currently registered by many different organisations, a situation that is confusing for those trying to find a reputable practitioner. There are umbrella organisations that attempt to unite the different registering

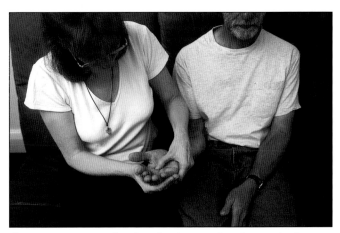

If necessary, massage can be adapted to the constraints of conventional healthcare settings by limiting work to the hands, head, or neck and shoulders

bodies in massage and aromatherapy but not in reflexology. It is probably wise to choose a practitioner from an organisation that is a member association of the British Complementary Medicine Association (BCMA) as these associations are regularly reviewed by the BCMA panel (see earlier article on complementary medicine in practice for contact details of BCMA).

Conventional healthcare professionals, who may have undertaken massage training but not have formal qualifications, are regulated by their own professional body.

Training
The variety of training courses is enormous, with many specifically aimed at conventional healthcare workers such as nurses. A central examinations agency, the International Therapy Examinations Council (ITEC), holds examinations in massage and related therapies that are accepted by many organisations. Other courses range from weekend courses in basic massage to university degree courses in therapeutic massage.

The pictures of full massage and of massage oil are reproduced with permission of Damien Lovegrove/Science Photo Library. The pictures of baby massage and hand massage are reproduced with permission of BMJ/Ulrike Preuss. The picture of massage in a hospital is reproduced with permission of the Royal London Homoeopathic Hospital. The picture of essential oils is reproduced with permission of Steve Horrell/Science Photo Library.

Umbrella organisations involved in registering massage based therapies

British Massage Therapy Council
17 Rymers Lane, Oxford OX4 3JU. Tel: 01865 774123 (for lists of registered practitioners 020 8992 2554). URL: www.bmtc.co.uk

Aromatherapy Organisations Council
PO Box 19834 London SE25 6WF. Tel: 020 8251 7912. Fax: 020 8251 7942. URL: www.aromatherapy-uk.org

Further reading

● Vickers A. *Massage and aromatherapy: a guide for health professionals.* Cheltenham: Stanley Thornes, 1998

10 Unconventional approaches to nutritional medicine

Although nutrition, as a science, has always been part of conventional medicine, doctors are not taught, and therefore do not practise, much in the way of nutritional therapeutics. Dieticians in conventional settings tend to work mainly with particular patient groups—such as those with diabetes, obesity, digestive or swallowing problems, or cardiovascular risk factors. Apart from the treatment of gross nutritional deficiencies and rare metabolic disorders, other nutritional interventions generally fall outside the mainstream and can therefore be described as complementary medicine.

Background

There is a wide spectrum of complementary nutritional practices. These range from specific, well researched, biochemically understood treatments that are given by well trained practitioners to unresearched, biochemically implausible interventions popularised by spectacular claims in the lay press and largely used without professional supervision.

Just which treatments are "conventional" and which are "complementary" is subject to debate. Some, such as fish oil supplements for patients with rheumatoid arthritis, have many of the features of a conventional medical treatment—a biochemical mechanism and support from randomised trials—but are, none the less, often considered unconventional. Other interventions were originally considered "complementary" but are now part of conventional practice. Probably the best example is the high fibre diet, rich in fruit and vegetables. "Alternative" practitioners of the 19th century, such as John Kellogg, advocated such a diet at a time when conventional nutritional authorities tended to see meat and potatoes as the best food, even to the extent of denigrating the importance of vegetables and describing wheat bran as "refuse."

Nutritional interventions

Unconventional nutritional interventions can be broadly divided into three categories: nutritional supplements, dietary modification, and therapeutic systems.

Nutritional supplements
As well as various vitamins and minerals, the range of nutritional supplements includes many animal and plant products. Some of these have known active ingredients, such as γ-linolenic acid in evening primrose oil. Others, such as blue-green algae and kelp, have not been fully characterised biochemically. Some supplements are taken to improve general health and performance, while others are for specific clinical indications. Most are taken in pill form. There is some overlap between herbal and nutritional supplements.

Dietary modification
This involves more comprehensive changes in eating patterns. Many diets, such as vegetarianism and veganism, originated as "movements" characterised by political and ecological concerns, a moral stance towards food, and a view of diet as inseparable from lifestyle. Many diets are based on theoretical considerations rather than empirical data. For example, the rationale for the Hay diet's principle that starch and protein

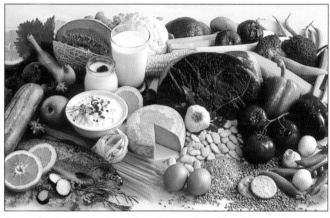

Conventional doctors only rarely make use of nutritional interventions, which is perhaps one reason why nutritional medicine has come to be regarded as part of complementary medicine

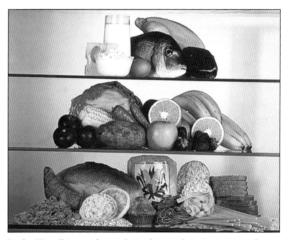

In the Hay diet proteins and starch must be eaten separately, though fruit and vegetables can be eaten with either

---

Examples of nutritional supplementation

- High dose vitamin C for cancer
- Zinc for the common cold
- High dose vitamins for learning disability ("orthomolecular" therapy)
- Evening primrose oil for atopic dermatitis
- Evening primrose oil for premenstrual syndrome
- Vitamin B-6 for morning sickness
- Vitamin B-6 for premenstrual syndrome
- Garlic for lowering cardiovascular risk
- Multivitamins for improvement in general health

Examples of diets claimed to improve general health

- Hay diet—Proteins and carbohydrates eaten separately
- Raw foods diet—Avoidance of cooked foods
- Stone Age diet—Avoids grains, pulses, and other products of the agricultural revolution
- Macrobiotic diet—Largely grains and vegetables. Foods are chosen and balanced in accordance with traditional oriental principles such as yin and yang
- Veganism—Avoids all animal products

---

should not be eaten together is that each type of food requires a different pH for optimum digestion. The principle of the Stone Age diet is that humans are not adapted by evolution to eat grains and pulses.

Therapeutic systems

These include techniques such as elimination dieting and naturopathy. Elimination dieting is based on the principle that foods particular to each patient may contribute to chronic symptoms or disease when eaten in normal quantities. Unlike classic allergy, these "food intolerances" do not involve a conventionally understood immune mechanism or inevitably have a rapid onset.

Diagnosis consists of eliminating all but a few foods from the diet and then reintroducing foods one by one to see if they provoke symptoms. After a period of complete exclusion, the problem substances can usually be gradually reintroduced without recurrence of symptoms. Although practitioners commonly diagnose wheat and dairy "intolerance," each patient is said to be sensitive to a different set of foods.

Naturopathy is a therapeutic system emphasising the philosophy of "nature cure" and incorporating dietary intervention among other practices such as hydrotherapy and exercise. For example, a naturopath might advise a patient with recurrent vaginal candidiasis to undertake a limited fast, reduce intake of foods containing sugar and yeast, and take herbal and probiotic preparations.

Another therapeutic system tests patients for "subclinical" nutritional deficiencies—thought to arise where systems of food intake, digestion, or absorption are not fully functional—and gives appropriate supplementation.

What happens during a treatment?

Many people make unconventional nutritional changes without consulting a practitioner (see below). Where practitioners are involved in treatment, consultations may involve some form of testing for deficiencies of particular nutrients or hidden allergies. Such tests include biochemical assays of the vitamin and mineral content of blood or hair. In "Vega" or electrodermal testing an electrical circuit is made that includes both the patient and the foodstuff suspected of causing disease. In applied kinesiology practitioners claim to be able to diagnose allergy or deficiency on the basis of changes in muscle function.

Evidence of therapeutic scope

Randomised controlled trials have favoured a small number of indications for high dose vitamin and mineral supplementation. These include both vitamin C and zinc for treating (though not for preventing) the common cold, vitamin B-6 for premenstrual syndrome (though trials are not of high quality) and autism, and vitamin E for angina.

There is evidence that exclusion dieting can be of benefit for various conditions including rheumatoid arthritis, hyperactivity, and migraine. However, only a minority of patients with such conditions seem to benefit, and it is not yet possible to select these in advance. Randomised trials have shown that increasing consumption of polyunsaturated fatty acids—for example, by supplementation with products such as fish oils or evening primrose oil—and reducing saturates can be beneficial in hypertriglyceridaemia, rheumatoid arthritis, and inflammatory bowel disease.

The evidence for most other unconventional nutritional interventions in treating disease is generally either negative or

---

Examples of dietary interventions claimed to help in specific conditions

- Dong diet for arthritis—Recommends a diet similar to that of Chinese peasants
- Feingold diet for attention deficit disorder—Recommends elimination of food additives
- Polyunsaturated fatty acid diet for multiple sclerosis
- Gluten-free diets for schizophrenia
- Atkins diet—Recommends elimination of all carbohydrates for weight loss
- "F-plan"—High fibre diet for weight loss
- Dairy-free diet for recurrent respiratory disease
- Gerson diet for cancer—Strictly vegetarian, largely raw food, diet with coffee enemas, and various supplements

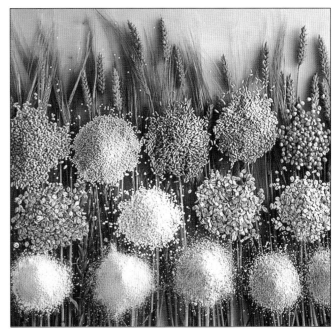

In the Stone Age diet grains, pulses, and other products of the agricultural revolution must be avoided. Such exclusion diets can be highly restrictive, socially disruptive, and expensive

---

Key studies of efficacy or reliability

Systematic reviews
- Douglas RM, Chalker EB, Treacy B. Vitamin C for the common cold. In: The Cochrane Collaboration. *The Cochrane Library*. Issue 2. Oxford: Update Software, 1998
- Fortin PR, Lew RA, Liang MH, Wright EA, Beckett LA, Chalmers TC, et al. Validation of a meta-analysis: the effects of fish oil in rheumatoid arthritis. *J Clin Epidemiol* 1995;48:1379-90
- Budeiri D, Li Wan Po A, Dornan JC. Is evening primrose oil of value in the treatment of premenstrual syndrome? *Controlled Clin Trials* 1996;17:60-8
- Wyatt KM, Dimmock PW, Jones PW, O'Brien PMS. Efficacy of vitamin B-6 in the treatment of premenstrual syndrome: systematic review. *BMJ* 1999;318:1375-81

Randomised controlled trial
- Schmidt MH, Mocks P, Lay B, Eisert HG, Fojkar R, Fritz Sigmund D, et al. Does oligoantigenic diet influence hyperactive/conduct-disordered children—a controlled trial. *Eur Child Adolesc Psychiatry* 1997;6:88-95

Study of reliability
- Sethi TJ, Kemeny DM, Tobin S, Lessof MH, Lambourn E, Bradley A. How reliable are commercial allergy tests? *Lancet* 1987;i:92-4

non-existent. For example, randomised trials have failed to show any benefit from high dose vitamin C for cancer; megadose therapy for Down's syndrome, learning disability, or schizophrenia; the Dong diet for arthritis; essential fatty acid supplementation for psoriasis or premenstrual syndrome; and vitamin B-6 for carpal tunnel syndrome.

Many unconventional diets are claimed to have benefits in specific conditions and general effects on physical health, mental wellbeing, and even spiritual development. Apart from those discussed above, these have not been evaluated systematically. There has been no rigorous research on the naturopathic approach to chronic disease or on individualised nutritional therapy.

Nutritional tests

While some unconventional laboratories use assays and methods of quality control similar to those used in mainstream biochemical laboratories, others may be less reliable.

In studies where duplicate samples of hair or blood were sent to "alternative" nutritional testing laboratories there was low agreement in results for the same individual. In one investigation several laboratories which advertise services to the general public failed to report fish allergy in subjects who were allergic to fish but ascribed numerous (but inconsistent) allergies to healthy controls.

There is insufficient evidence on the validity of "Vega" testing. Studies have also found that practitioners of techniques such as applied kinesiology are unable to obtain consistent results from duplicate blinded samples.

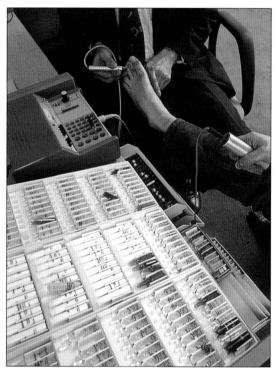

Vega testing is said to identify patients' individual food intolerances. Although its validity remains uncertain, it is often used to draw up personalised elimination diet programmes

Safety

Most unconventional diets recommend generally healthy patterns of eating (reduction or elimination of fat, sugar, alcohol, and coffee and an increase in fresh vegetables and fibre) which most people with a normal digestion can tolerate without side effects.

Some diets, such as veganism or macrobiotics, are highly restrictive and can lead to complications such as reduced bone mass or anaemia, especially in children. Children, pregnant and lactating women, and patients with chronic illness should undertake such major dietary changes only under professional supervision. A drawback of any dietary change can be social disruption when a patient cannot share meals with friends and family.

High dose nutritional supplementation can lead to acute adverse effects such as diarrhoea (vitamin C) and flushing (niacin) during treatment. Persistent or more serious adverse effects are rare for water soluble vitamins, although chronic use of high dose vitamin B-6 can lead to neuropathies. Adverse effects, though still uncommon, are more likely to result from high doses of fat soluble vitamins: vitamin A has been linked with birth defects and irreversible bone and liver damage, and vitamin D with hypercalcaemia. High doses of single minerals or amino acids may induce deficiency in nutrients that share similar metabolic pathways. Excessive doses of zinc and selenium can cause immune suppression, and evening primrose oil may exacerbate temporal lobe epilepsy.

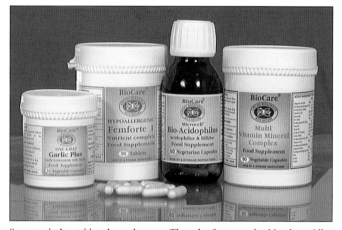

Some typical nutritional supplements. Though often perceived by the public to be inherently safe, supplements can sometimes be associated with adverse effects, especially when taken in high doses for long periods

Practice

Decisions to make unconventional nutritional changes are reached by many routes, often through the use of self help books, leaflets, and magazine articles or advice from friends, relatives, and staff of health food stores. People may also make

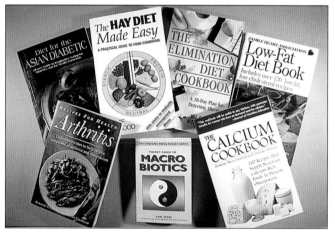

Many patients undertake unconventional diets without advice from a practitioner of any kind

changes on the basis of nutritional tests provided by commercial companies which advertise laboratory services in the pages of health magazines.

Nutritional consultations may be given by a wide range of practitioners with varying levels of training and experience, from complementary practitioners who mainly practise other disciplines through trained nutritional therapists and naturopaths to nurses and doctors who have undertaken further training in nutrition.

Nutritional medicine can be a relatively expensive form of complementary medicine. Diagnostic tests can cost from £15 to over £100 per test, nutritional supplements may cost £10-£50 a month, and dietary changes involving organic produce or wholefoods may also have substantial cost implications.

Regulation

The General Council and Register of Naturopaths registers and regulates the 180 or so naturopaths practising in the United Kingdom. Most of these are also trained osteopaths. Regulation for other nutritional practitioners is not as well established. The British Association of Nutritional Therapists registers and arranges mandatory insurance for about 200 practitioners who have completed one of the more thorough courses at selected training colleges. A few smaller registers also exist.

Training

Various courses in nutritional therapy exist, ranging from short courses of a few days leading to a certificate in basic nutrition to three year, part time courses leading to qualification as a nutritional therapist. Naturopaths in Britain usually undergo a four year, full time training which includes anatomy, physiology, biochemistry, and pathology as well as naturopathic and osteopathic principles and practice.

The British Society for Allergy, Environmental, and Nutritional Medicine is an association of doctors with a special interest in nutrition. It organises educational events and publishes the *Journal of Nutritional and Environmental Medicine*.

Regulatory bodies in nutritional medicine

General Council and Register of Naturopaths
2 Goswell Road, Street, Somerset BA16 0JG. Tel: 01458 840072. Fax: 01458 840075. Email: admin@naturopathy.org.uk. URL: www.naturopathy.org.uk

British Association of Nutritional Therapists
BCM BANT, London WC1N 3XX. Tel: 0870 606 1284

Training and educational organisations

Department of Nutritional Medicine, University of Surrey
Offers part time postgraduate courses up to MSc level aimed at doctors, dieticians and nutritional therapists
c/o Course Administrator for Nutritional Medicine School of Biological Sciences, University of Surrey, Guildford, Surrey GU2 5XH. Tel: 01483 876465. Fax: 01483 876481. URL: www.surrey.ac.uk (access via biological sciences)

British Society for Allergy, Environmental and Nutritional Medicine (BSAENM)
Membership organisation for doctors only
For publications: PO Box 28, Totton, Southampton SO40 2ZA. Tel: 023 80812124
For inquiries: PO Box 7, Knighton LD7 1WT. Tel: Premierline 0906 3020010

Further reading

- Anthony H, Birtwhistle S, Eaton K, Maberly J. *Environmental medicine in clinical practice.* Southampton: BSAENM Publications, 1997
- Brostoff J, Gamlin L. *Complete guide to food allergy and intolerance.* London: Bloomsbury, 1992
- Davies S, Stewart A. *Nutritional medicine.* London: Pan, 1987
- Murray M, Pizzorno J. *Encyclopaedia of natural medicine.* 2nd ed. London: Little, Brown, 1999

11 Complementary medicine and the patient

In surveys of users of complementary medicine, about 80% are satisfied with the treatment they received. Interestingly, this is not always dependent on an improvement in their presenting complaint. For example, in one UK survey of cancer patients, changes attributed to complementary medicine included being emotionally stronger, less anxious, and more hopeful about the future even if the cancer remained unchanged.

Satisfaction may influence further use of complementary medicine: a Community Health Council survey found that over two thirds of complementary medicine users returned for further courses of treatment and that over 90% thought that they might use complementary medicine in the future. What is it that patients find worth while and what does this tell us about their expectations of healthcare services in general?

Attraction of complementary medicine

The specific effects of particular therapies obviously account for a proportion of patient satisfaction, but surveys and qualitative research show that many patients also value some of the general attributes of complementary medicine. These may include the relationship with their practitioner, the ways in which illness is explained, and the environment in which they receive treatment. When these augment the therapeutic outcome of treatment, they contribute to what is sometimes called "the placebo effect." None of these is unique to complementary medicine, but many are facilitated by the private, non-institutional settings in which most complementary practitioners work. The relative therapeutic importance of specific and non-specific attributes obviously depends on individual patients and practitioners, but some complementary practitioners may be better than their conventional colleagues at using and maximising "the placebo effect."

Time and continuity
Patients often cite the amount of time available for consultation as a reason for choosing complementary medicine, and contrast this with their experiences of seeing conventional NHS doctors. This is partly a feature of all private medicine, but even when complementary practitioners work in the NHS their first appointments tend to be up to an hour long in order to take the detailed case history that diagnosis and treatment requires.

Particularly when the problem is chronic and multifactorial, this type of consultation, in which patients are encouraged to explain their experience and understanding of their problem, can itself be therapeutic. Patients also generally see the same complementary practitioner over their course of treatment, and this continuity further facilitates the development of a therapeutic patient-practitioner relationship.

Attention to personality and personal experience
All healthcare practitioners, conventional or complementary, aim to tailor their interventions to the needs of individual patients. However, conventional practitioners generally direct treatment at the underlying disease processes, whereas many complementary practitioners base treatment more on the way patients experience and manifest their disease, including their psychology and response to illness. Treatment is

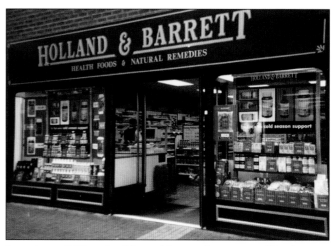

Increasing availability of and demand for complementary medicine is evidence of its popularity. The question is whether this represents a passing fashion or a deeper need for change within the healthcare system

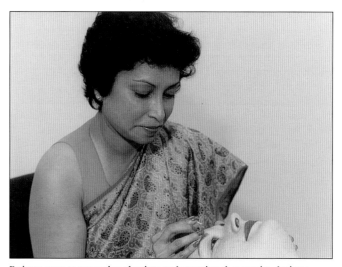

Patients seem to appreciate the time and attention they receive during a complementary medicine consultation

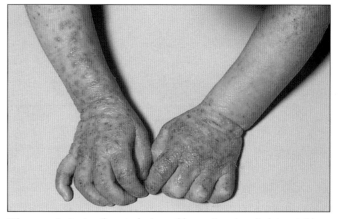

Whereas a doctor treating atopic dermatitis may be primarily interested in the condition of the skin, complementary practitioners often take as much account of personality and emotions as they do of physical signs and symptoms

"individualised" in both cases, but patients' personalities and emotions may be more influential in the latter approach.

Although good conventional care involves considering the patient as a person, not a disease, time pressures can lead to an apparent emphasis on the physical aspects of illness. Some patients cite the lack of personal attention paid by conventional practitioners as a reason for choosing a complementary approach. The quality of personal attention is obviously influenced by time and continuity as described above.

Patient involvement and choice
Some users cite the increased opportunities for active participation in the process of recovery as a reason for choosing complementary medicine. Although self help measures are increasingly part of conventional healthcare advice, patients feel that complementary practitioners give this greater emphasis.

Patients also value being able to choose a complementary therapist or therapy which suits them. To some extent, this is true of all private sector health care, but it is also possible when a choice of different complementary approaches is available on the NHS. An example would be the range of complementary therapies available in many hospices.

Hope
Patients often come to complementary medicine after having tried everything that conventional medicine has to offer. Complementary practitioners can offer hope to such patients, both by attempting to influence the underlying disease and, often more importantly, by addressing emotional states, energy levels, coping styles, and other aspects that contribute to quality of life. This is particularly important for patients with chronic diseases and no prospect of cure from conventional medicine. However, practitioners need to balance their claims carefully, considering the realistic chances of improvement and the dangers of creating false hope and further disappointment.

Touch
Many complementary treatments and diagnostic techniques involve more physical contact between patients and practitioners than is usual in conventional medicine. Touch can facilitate more open and honest communication, and patients may turn to the "low tech" consulting rooms of aromatherapists and reflexologists for a less distancing and more human experience of health care.

Dealing with ill defined symptoms
Practitioners of modern Western medicine have become expert in recognising, identifying, and treating disease. When there is no organic disease present but simply ill defined symptoms or a general "lack of health" they may have less to offer. As a result, patients presenting with illnesses such as chronic fatigue, functional back pain, or irritable bowel syndrome may feel that their doctor does not take their symptoms seriously or does not really believe that they are ill. Complementary practitioners do not need a conventional diagnosis to initiate treatment; in fact, many think that their treatments are most effective in patients without organic pathology. (The risks of missing serious conditions if complementary treatments are given to patients without definite diagnoses are considered in the next article.)

Making sense of illness
Patients often want to incorporate their experience of illness into their understanding of themselves and their world. They ask questions like "Why has this happened to me?" and "What in my life has caused my problem?" Complementary practitioners may have explanations that make sense to

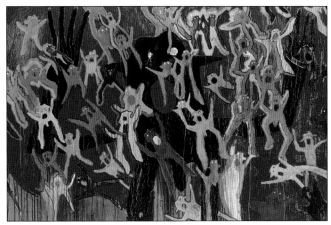
"Prostate Roar" by Ian Summers (1998), painted during art therapy after his prostate cancer had been diagnosed. Art therapy, like many complementary therapies, can help patients to construct a meaningful narrative of disease

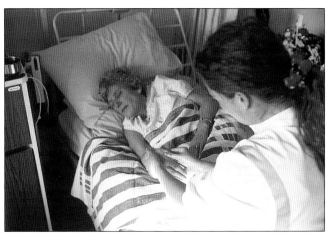
Aromatherapy massage in a hospice. Many forms of complementary medicine involve physical contact with patients

Attitudes to touch through massage
Staff member in learning difficulties unit—"People with profound disabilities often become isolated from any special caring touch. It's inappropriate for us to go around hugging and cuddling pupils, but we can use hand and foot massage"

Cancer patient—"They're too busy, the nurses, ... rushing round the wards .... With massage, as soon as the hands go on, you know she's there, she's calm, she's touching you, she has time for you"

Patient in primary care—"Touch had never been common in my family. Massage has been complementary in giving me a structured experience of touch. The main benefit, though, was relearning to be at ease with my body, relax my mind, without being overcome with weeping or anxieties"

Example of a complementary practitioner's view of illness
A patient with chronic ear infections consulted a complementary practitioner, who associated his problem with bad dietary habits and longstanding digestive problems:

"She said that, from a holistic point of view, if you cannot eliminate in the normal way, where does the residual muck go? It can go into your eyes, your breath, and your ears. And, lo and behold, I realised it. She said I was excreting rubbish through my ears, and this, of course, fitted into place, because it was black and sticky. No one ever told me that; they just said, 'You're producing too much wax' "

Taken from Sharma 1995

patients—such as describing illness as a result of environmental factors or as a physical expression of emotional patterns.

Conventional medicine may have problems with such explanations if they have no scientific justification, but sociological research shows that patients consider them beneficial when they reinforce their own beliefs and expectations. Sometimes the explanations given by complementary practitioners can cause problems—for example, if illness is attributed to childhood vaccinations or patients are made to feel guilty for past behaviour.

Spiritual and existential concerns
Some patients have existential concerns that conventionally trained professionals may not feel competent to address. These range from the otherwise healthy adolescent who can find no meaning or purpose in life to the terminally ill patient confronting his or her own mortality. Many complementary disciplines make no distinction between spiritual symptoms and any other types of symptom and offer treatments aimed at this aspect of a person's life or illness.

Concern over complementary medicine

The general attributes of complementary medicine do not always lead to increased patient satisfaction. Complementary medicine has some features that can cause patients problems or produce negative effects. Those that primarily involve patients' practical or emotional responses are described below. Those that may pose risks to patients' overall healthcare are covered in the next article.

Safety and competence
There is public anxiety that some complementary practitioners may not be adequately qualified, although patients who have already used complementary medicine show less concern. Patients' inability to trust in the competence of their complementary practitioner will influence their experience of treatment. The lack of nationally recognised professional standards for some therapies is a major problem.

Patients often make assumptions about the safety of complementary medication bought over the counter. As many of these contain pharmacologically active agents, they have the potential for adverse effects, particularly where they are taken in combination with other complementary or conventional medication.

Guilt
One potential danger of empowering patients to play an active part in improving their health is that some come to believe that they are solely responsible for their ill health or lack of recovery. For example, patients who are encouraged to take a positive attitude in fighting cancer can suffer increased distress if they infer that their illness is a product of an excessively negative personality. Complementary practitioners need to be aware of this potential when giving advice and explanations to vulnerable patients.

Denial
Some patients continue to try different complementary therapies even though none has given any relief. This behaviour can promote an unhelpful pattern of denial about a condition. Repeated attempts to find a cure through complementary medicine can prevent appropriate acceptance and adjustment.

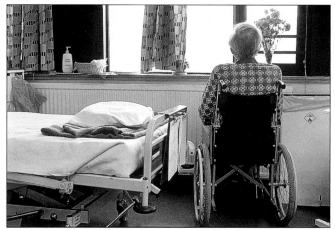

Conventional medicine may leave patients' spiritual and existential concerns unmet

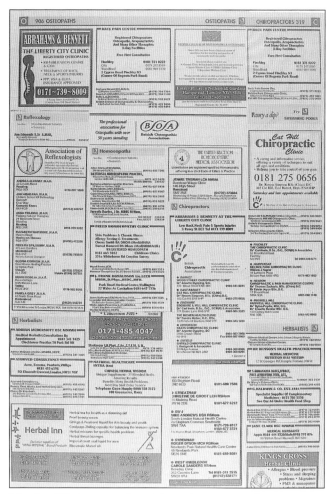

It is often difficult to assess the training and competence of complementary practitioners

---

Potential for inducing guilt and blame in complementary medicine literature
Louise Hay—"All disease comes from a state of unforgiveness"
Edward Bach—"Rigidity of mind will give rise to those diseases which produce rigidity and stiffness of the body"
Alexander Lowen—"A weakness in the backbone must be reflected in serious personality disturbance … the individual with sway back cannot have the ego strength of a person whose back is straight"

Complementary practitioners need to be aware of the risks of colluding with this behaviour.

Blame

Some of the explanations given by complementary practitioners emphasise external and environmental causes of illness. For example, they may claim a disease is caused by vaccinations, conventional drugs, drinking water, dental fillings, or pollution. Placing the blame for ill health solely on external factors that cannot easily be altered may lead to patients feeling victimised, disempowered, and bitter. There may be other factors influencing their illness, and helpful coping strategies, that could be more usefully addressed.

Financial risk

The amount of money some patients spend on complementary medicine is considerable. Costs vary widely, and higher prices do not necessarily mean better or more effective treatment. The lack of evidence concerning many complementary interventions means that the likelihood of a successful outcome is often impossible to predict. Patients should be aware of this risk. They should also be encouraged to ask practitioners, and seek guidance from the main regulatory bodies, about estimated costs for a complete course of treatment, including tests and medications, before starting complementary therapy.

Social factors

Most users of complementary medicine in Britain are of middle to high socioeconomic status. Possibly as a result, the effects of poverty, poor housing, and discrimination are underplayed in complementary accounts of disease causation.

Further reading

- Benson H. *Timeless healing; the power and biology of belief.* London: Simon and Schuster 1996
- Bishop B. *A time to heal.* 2nd ed. London: Arkana, 1996
- Sharma U. *Complementary medicine today: practitioners and patients.* Rev ed. London: Routledge, 1995

The picture of a health food shop is reproduced with permission of Holland and Barrett. The picture of acupuncture is reproduced with permission of the Royal London Homoeopathic Hospital. The picture of eczematous hands is reproduced with permission of the National Medical Slide Bank. "Prostate Roar" is reproduced with permission of the University of Pennsylvania Cancer Center. The picture of aromatherapy is reproduced with permission of John Cole/ Impact. The picture of a hospital patient is reproduced with permission of Tony Stone Images/Adam Hinton.

12 Complementary medicine and the doctor

Doctors deal with complementary medicine in a variety of professional situations. Patients may ask for advice about whether to pursue complementary therapies or which therapist to consult; they may request referral or delegation, either privately or on the NHS; or they may want to discuss treatment or advice given by complementary practitioners. Doctors prescribing drugs to patients taking complementary treatments may have concerns about possible interactions. Doctors should therefore consider strategies for minimising risk and facilitating sensible and appropriate discussions with patients and complementary practitioners.

Medical attitudes

Surveys of doctors' attitudes to complementary medicine show that, overall, physicians believe it is moderately effective, but low response rates make some studies unreliable. Although hospital doctors and older general practitioners tend to be more sceptical than younger doctors and medical students, most respondents believe that some of the more established forms are of benefit and should be available on the NHS. Younger doctors and medical students are more likely to perceive their knowledge of complementary medicine as inadequate and to want more tuition in the subject.

Qualitative research shows that many doctors want to be supportive of patients' choices and would welcome further information, although they generally regard complementary therapies as scientifically unproved. Doctors' concerns about such therapies include whether they are used as an adjunct or an alternative to conventional care, how effective conventional treatments are in the given condition, and the possibility of adverse effects.

Promoting good practice

Doctors can have an important role in identifying patients who use complementary medicine, minimising their risk of harm, and, as far as possible, ensuring that their choice of treatment is in their best interests. The key to achieving this in practice is often to maintain open, clear, and effective communication with patients, and sometimes complementary practitioners.

Identifying complementary medicine users
There is evidence that most people who have used complementary medicine do not tell their doctors. Specific questions may be required to elicit use, as when inquiring about drugs and alcohol intake.

Minimising potential risks
As discussed in earlier articles, there are potential risks associated with the use of complementary medicine. Although these are likely to be rare, it is important that patients are adequately informed and take basic precautions to reduce their chances of harm.

Delayed or missed diagnosis
Many conventional professionals are concerned that, if complementary treatments are given to patients before a definite diagnosis has been made, serious pathology and

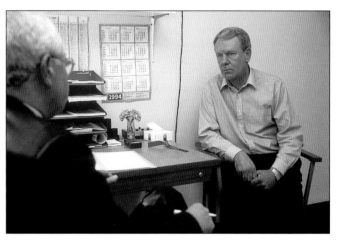

Most patients do not tell their general practitioner if they are using complementary medicine. This may place some at unnecessary risk

---

Common concerns of doctors about complementary medicine
- Patients may see unqualified complementary practitioners
- Patients may risk missed or delayed diagnosis
- Patients may stop or refuse effective conventional treatment
- Patients may waste money on ineffective treatments
- Patients may experience dangerous adverse effects from treatment
- The mechanism of some complementary treatments is so implausible they cannot possibly work

---

Consider asking about complementary medicine use when
- Patient has chronic or relapsing disease
- Conventional approaches require maintenance treatment
- Patient is experiencing or is concerned about adverse drug reactions
- Patient is unhappy about progress
- There is unexplained poor compliance with treatment or follow up

---

Useful questions when inquiring about use of complementary medicine

Healthcare behaviour
- Have you tried any other treatment approaches for this problem?
- Have you ever seen a complementary or alternative practitioner for this problem?
- Have you ever tried changing your diet because you thought it might help this problem?
- Have you used any herbal or natural remedies that you have bought from a chemist or health food shop?

Healthcare attitudes
- What are you hoping will come out of your complementary treatment?
- What was it that encouraged you to try complementary medicine?

Communication and cooperation
- Would you like to ask your complementary therapist to let me know about your treatment and progress?

opportunities for effective conventional treatment may be missed. This is a real concern; there are a few reports of fatalities occurring for this reason. However, evidence indicates that most patients with ongoing symptoms consult their general practitioners before trying complementary medicine.

In addition, practitioner members of the main complementary medicine regulatory bodies are usually trained to recognise "red flag" symptoms and redirect patients to conventional care. For example, there are reports of chiropractors and osteopaths diagnosing spinal malignancies and referring appropriately. Problems are less likely if patients are using complementary medicine alongside conventional care. Doctors and complementary practitioners both have a role in ensuring that patients seek medical assessment and follow up before, during, and after complementary treatment for persisting problems.

Stopping or refusing conventional care

There are reports of serious adverse consequences of complementary practitioners giving advice which contradicts that of a doctor. Most of these occur because patients suddenly stop beneficial maintenance medication such as asthma or anticonvulsant treatment. Immunisations, antibiotics, and diet are other areas where the influence of complementary medicine can cause particular difficulties. Again, good communication between all parties is the most effective protection, and patients should be made aware of the risks of sudden changes. Patients taking long term medication should be encouraged to find a complementary practitioner who is happy to liaise and cooperate with their general practitioner.

Interaction between complementary and conventional treatments

Little information has been published on the combined use of complementary and conventional treatments, but some serious interactions have been reported. These have mostly involved herbal products or dietary supplements. The lack of a formal reporting system makes their true incidence unknown, and more reliable information is needed. Encouraging patients who are taking conventional medication to disclose and discuss intentions to use complementary therapies, and to initiate treatment only under medical supervision, may help to reduce risks.

Preventing fragmentation of care

Use of complementary medicine is not generally recorded in general practitioners' notes. A patient's health care may therefore become fragmented and uncoordinated. Again, good communication between complementary practitioners and general practitioners can greatly improve this situation.

Finding a reputable practitioner

Patients should be encouraged to follow a few simple rules when choosing a complementary practitioner (see box).

Knowing what to expect

Increased awareness of some of the general problems that can occur with complementary treatment and the specific adverse effects of the individual therapies (see earlier articles) can help patients make more informed choices.

Ensuring treatment is in the patient's best interests

Although most patients seek complementary medicine on quite reasonable grounds, there are cases when a patient's use of complementary treatments should be questioned.

Essentials of good practice in complementary medicine

- The practitioner should practise only to the level to which he or she has achieved competence
- The practitioner should take a sufficient medical history to ensure there are no contraindications to the intended treatment
- The practitioner should not advise any changes to conventional treatment without seeking the advice of a doctor
- The practitioner should ideally communicate with the patient's general practitioner, including the following information: complementary medicine diagnosis, all treatment and advice given, likely duration of treatment, date of discharge or any follow up plans
- There should an agreed time frame in which progress should be assessed

---

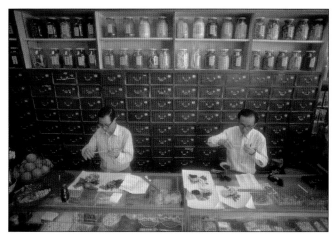

A Chinese herbal pharmacy. As many complementary medicines contain pharmacologically active agents it is important to establish what patients are using in order to minimise the risk of interactions with conventional drugs

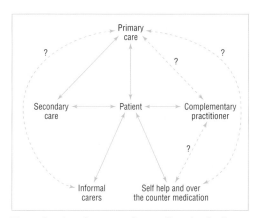

The patient is at the centre of a complicated web of healthcare activity and communication: the use of complementary medicine may increase the potential for fragmented care

---

Finding a reputable complementary medicine practitioner

- The practitioner should have current registration and follow the code of conduct laid out by the appropriate complementary medicine professional body
- The practitioner should hold full insurance to practise in the relevant setting (employers or regular referrers should ask to see current insurance certificates)
- In addition, references from a respected and impartial third party (such as a previous client, NHS employer, etc) may be sought

Patient has unrealistic expectations

High expectations can be generated or encouraged by complementary practitioners and sensational media coverage. However, they are often a feature of a patient's unwillingness to accept a diagnosis of chronic or progressive disease.

Costs outweigh the benefits

Patients often seek complementary medicine for longstanding and difficult to manage problems. In order to maintain hope of improvement or cure they may continue to pay for treatment long after it has become clear that it is not of value. The lack of routine assessments or incentives for private practitioners to bring treatment to an end may exacerbate this situation. Patients may sometimes feel guilty about lack of progress and find it difficult to stop seeing a complementary practitioner. Most reputable practitioners assess progress regularly with their patients.

Taking patients seriously

Patients who are considering complementary medicine may have underlying motives that need exploration. Discussing these fully with a doctor may be therapeutic, and sometimes sufficient in itself. Patients may be experiencing unacceptable side effects from conventional treatment or have difficulty adjusting to their illness. While doctors cannot be expected to provide detailed advice about complementary treatments, they should be aware of their patients' health concerns and beliefs. A doctor who listens and supports patient choice, and whose advice minimises risk, rather than dismisses complementary medicine on principle is more likely to encourage patients to use it appropriately, as an adjunct rather than an alternative to conventional care.

Facilitating effective communication

This article has stressed the need for effective communication between doctors, patients and complementary practitioners. There are, however, often considerable barriers to such communication. These may result from philosophical and cultural differences, private versus NHS settings, and from underlying issues of power and control. Practitioners should be aware that they may not all speak the same healthcare "language" or be looking for the same type of patient response. Written referral and discharge letters, discussions about individual patients, and multidisciplinary meetings can be helpful strategies.

Which therapy and which practitioner?

Doctors are used to a one to one correspondence between particular diseases and particular treatments. Many complementary techniques, however, have broad and overlapping indications. For example, evidence shows that acupuncture can treat conditions as disparate as stroke, nausea, and chronic pain and that pain can respond to treatments as disparate as acupuncture, manipulation, and hypnosis.

Determining the most appropriate therapy for an individual patient is therefore generally a case of identifying those techniques for which there is the strongest evidence of benefit in the given condition and choosing the one that the patient finds most acceptable and believes is most likely to be of benefit. Finding the right practitioner—one who is appropriately qualified, with whom the patient and doctor can communicate and trust—is a prime consideration.

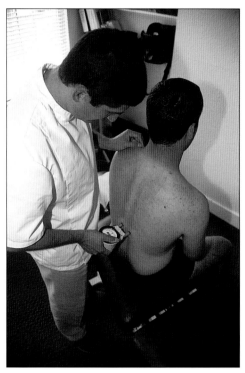

Reputable complementary practitioners should regularly assess progress with their patients

Dealing with interdisciplinary issues with complementary practitioners

- Encourage patients to voice their concerns
- Refrain from personally directed criticism of other practitioners
- Offer your professional opinion neutrally
- Offer patients a chance for a second opinion
- If malpractice or abuse is suspected, obtain as much information as possible to support your position and seek advice from your defence society and from the relevant complementary medicine professional body

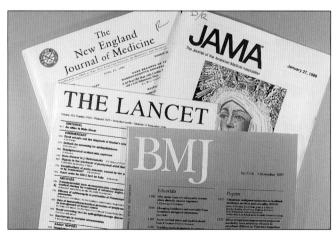

Although doctors may claim to be unaware of published data on complementary medicine, results from many randomised controlled trials of complementary medicine have been published in major, peer reviewed journals

Learning about complementary medicine

It has been argued that doctors should learn about complementary medicine because it is widely used and because it may have substantial beneficial and harmful effects. Informal methods of education—such as reading books or journals, searching the internet, or via contact with practitioners or practitioner organisations—are not always objective or reliable. The BMA recommends establishing more formal "familiarisation" initiatives.

Nearly half of all UK medical schools now offer limited teaching in complementary medicine, although standards vary and courses are usually an option for only a few students. Some postgraduate medical centres run courses of varying content and quality that are approved for postgraduate education allowance to provide a basic introduction to several complementary disciplines.

Some doctors undertake training to enable them to practise some form of complementary therapy. The basic choice is between courses that train non-medically qualified practitioners and those specifically designed for doctors. The former take considerably more time and involve a more detailed study of traditional techniques; the latter are shorter and often take a "medicalised" view of the complementary technique. Doctors may decide to learn a few simple techniques or to change their practice more fundamentally to specialise in a complementary discipline.

The picture of a general practice consultation is reproduced with permission of Antonia Reeve/Science Photo Library. The picture of a Chinese herbal pharmacy is reproduced with permission of Phil Schermeister/Corbis. The pictures of a chiropractic assessment and of medical journals are reproduced with permission of *BMJ*/Ulrike Preuss.

For their assistance with photographs used to illustrate this series, we thank Dr Carl D Irwin, chiropractic; Jill Hedison, osteopathy; David Charlaff, acupuncture; Roxanne Clark, massage; Carol Taylor, reflexology. We also thank Dr Sadeem Abutrab, Cassandra Marks, Helen Robertson, and Harrison Smith.

Sources of further information

General databases
- Medline—Includes some published research on complementary medicine, including papers from some specialist complementary medicine journals
- *Cochrane Library*—Includes most published controlled trials of complementary medicine. Search using the keyword "compmed"

Complementary medicine registering bodies
Hold codes of conduct, details of insurance cover, and lists of contraindications for most therapies
See earlier articles for full lists and addresses

Information on safety issues
See earlier articles about individual therapies

Information on the internet and email
- US National Institute of Health National Center for Complementary and Alternative Medicine (formerly Office of Alternative Medicine). URL: http://nccam.nih.gov
- Focus on Alternative and Complementary Medicine. URL: www.exeter.ac.uk/FACT
- Research Council for Complementary Medicine. Email: info@rccm.org.uk
See earlier articles for details about individual therapies

Further reading
- Lewith G, Kenyon J, Lewis P. *Complementary medicine: an integrated approach.* Oxford: Oxford University Press, 1996. (Oxford General Practice Series)
- Sharma U. *Complementary medicine today: practitioners and patients.* Rev ed. London: Routledge, 1995
- *Complementary medicine: new approaches to good practice.* Oxford: Oxford University Press, 1993
- Vincent C, Furnham A. Complementary medicine and the medical profession. In: *Complimentary medicine: a research perspective.* Chichester: John Wiley & Sons, 1997, pp 71- 75

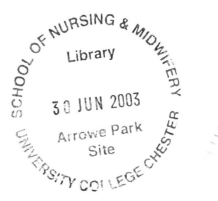

Index

Page numbers in bold refer to illustrations

Titles in the ABC series from BMJ Books

ABC of Labour Care
G Chamberlain, P Steer and L Zander

ABC of Major Trauma (3rd edition)
Edited by David Skinner and Peter Driscoll

ABC of Medical Computing
Nicholas Lee and Andrew Millman

ABC of Mental Health
Edited by Teifion Davies and T K J Craig

ABC of Monitoring Drug Therapy
J K Aronson, M Hardman and D J M Reynolds

ABC of Nutrition (3rd edition)
A Stewart Truswell

ABC of One to Seven (4th edition)
H B Valman

ABC of Otolaryngology (4th edition)
Harold Ludman

ABC of Palliative Care
Edited by Marie Fallon and Bill O'Neill

ABC of Resuscitation (4th edition)
Edited by M C Colquhoun, A J Handley and T R Evans

ABC of Rheumatology (2nd edition)
Edited by Michael L Snaith

ABC of Sexual Health
Edited by John Tomlinson

ABC of Sexually Transmitted Diseases (4th edition)
Michael W Adler

ABC of Spinal Cord Injury (3rd edition)
David Grundy and Andrew Swain

ABC of Sports Medicine (2nd edition)
Edited by G McLatchie, M Harries, C Williams and J King

ABC of Transfusion (3rd edition)
Edited by Marcela A Contreras

ABC of Urology
Chris Dawson and Hugh Whitfield

ABC of Vascular Diseases
Edited by John Wolfe

ABC of Work Related Disorders
Edited by David Snashall

The First Year of Life (4th edition)
H B Valman

To order, please contact BMJ Bookshop, PO Box 295, London WC1H 9TE, UK
Tel: +44 (0)20 7383 6244   **Fax**: +44 (0)20 7383 6455   **Email**: orders@bmjbookshop.com